# WRITE IT:

## THE NRMP PERSONAL STATEMENT WORKBOOK

Myers R. Hurt III, MD

ISBN: 978-0-9975955-3-6 (Print)
ISBN: 978-0-9975955-2-9 (E-version)

Editing and Proofing by Erika's Editing
Cover Design and Interior Formatting by Book Formatters

*To my former, current, and future medical students:*
*You will all make incredible physicians.*

# CONTENTS

**Introduction**     **1**

**Chapter 1: The Importance of Your Statement**     **5**
Understanding the Weight of Your Statement     5
Standing Out in a Sea of Candidates     7
Fleshing Out Your Qualifications     8
Showing Your Personality     9

**Chapter 2: General Guidelines for Your Statement**     **11**
The MyERAS Web Portal: Requirements and Tips     11
Common Pitfalls     13
Time Management: Protecting Your Writing Time     16

**Chapter 3: Brainstorming (Pre-writing, Part I)**     **19**
Creating Your Idea Cloud     20
Step 1: Seeding Your Cloud     21
     A Note on Your Statement and Red Flags     22
Step 2: Identify Your Strongest Ideas Using a Traits List     24
Step 3: Describe Your Specialty     26
Step 4: Relate Your Experiences to Your Specialty     28
Step 5: Rank the Best of the Best     30

**Chapter 4: Creative Writing 101 (Pre-writing, Part II)**     **33**
Show, Don't Tell     34
Storytelling Within an Essay Format     39
Striking the Right Tone     42
Building a Personal Brand     44

**Chapter 5: Writing Your First Draft**     **47**
Using the Active Voice     48
Strengthening Your Focus     49

Putting Pen to Paper                                      50
    A Note on Writing an Outline                          50
    Breaking Convention in Case of Emergency              52

**Chapter 6: Your Second and Third Drafts (Editing, Part I)    55**
Reviewing Your Statement                                  56
    A Tip for Tracking Your Edits                         57
Spot-Checking, Eight Essentials                           57
Examining the Mechanics of Your Writing                   61
Selecting Beta Readers and Asking for Feedback            68

**Chapter 7: Polishing Your Statement (Editing, Part II)    71**
Checking Your Grammar and Spelling                        71
Using Grammar and Spelling Tools                          73
Reading Your Work Out Loud                                76
Hiring a Professional Editor                              77
    A Few Words of Advice on Using Freelancing
    Marketplaces                                          79
**Chapter 8: Tailoring Your Statement and Uploading It
    to MyERAS                                             83**
The Benefits of Custom-Tailoring Your Statement           83
Tailoring Points                                          85
Micro-Tailoring                                           86
One Last Check                                            87
Submitting Your Statement via MyERAS                      88

**A Clean Bill of Health: (A Farewell from the Author)      91**

**Glossary of Specialized Acronyms & Terms                  93**

**Acknowledgments                                           95**

**About the Author                                          97**

# INTRODUCTION

Congratulations! You've made it through undergrad, you've been accepted to med school, you have two full years of medical study under your belt, and you're now in the middle of your clerkships. These are huge accomplishments, and earning your MD isn't far off. Now it's time for the next step in your journey: applying for residencies.

Your ERAS residency application will include many components, most of which are qualitatively based. But there's one part of your package that's inherently different from all the other components: your personal statement. In my experience, I've found that writing this statement is the toughest (and often the most dreaded) part of the application process for many students. It doesn't have to be: I'm here to ease your fears and guide you through the writing process.

Your passion is medicine, which means—among many other things—that you probably don't think of yourself as a writer. The idea of summing up your goals, strengths, and experiences in a few short essay pages is daunting. And, especially if you have strong USMLE scores, solid research to your name, and great letters of recommendation, an essay may even seem unnecessary. After all, you obviously worked hard to make it to this point. Shouldn't your achievements speak for themselves?

Surprisingly, the answer is no. In *Write It*, I'll explain why personal statements *matter now more than ever*, and I'll discuss how they can make the difference between Matching in your first- or second-choice program or finding yourself scrubbing into SOAP, where you'll be forced to scramble for any available residency regardless of your preferred specialization.

What makes me an expert on personal residency statements? Over the last five years, I've read thousands of statements for healthcare professionals. While I was on the faculty of UTMB-Galveston, part of my job was to assist students with their statements. Now that I'm in private practice, helping med students Match successfully remains a passion of mine. My first book, *Getting In*, which focuses on the residency interview process, is an Amazon bestseller. My podcast, "Countdown to the MATCH," has been downloaded over twenty thousand times across various platforms. *Write It* is another step on my journey of reaching out to emerging doctors.

I'm not the only one offering advice to residents, but—as you probably know all too well—most books aimed at med students tend to be expensive and dense. By contrast, this workbook is a practical, streamlined, inexpensive tool for writing a statement that will get *you* noticed by program directors. Without bogging you down with unnecessary information, as you read along, I'll also offer you a few pointers on using the ERAS application portal (MyERAS).

Writing a stellar statement doesn't require being a great writer. In this workbook, I'll explain how to brainstorm, write, draft, edit, and polish your statement until it reflects you at your very best and complements the rest of your application. We'll go step-by-step together; by following my proven method and breaking the writing process down into manageable pieces you'll be able to craft your essay in an exciting, engaging, attention-grabbing way.

The targeted writing exercises in this workbook employ a "learn by doing" approach. You'll read a section, then do the exercise for that section. This will encourage you to physically put this book down, spend some time reflecting, and then write your thoughts out. I'll offer you planning ideas, organizational methods, and language-usage tips that will shape your mindset as you go through the chapters.

Yes, you read that right: I said read a section, then do the exercises for that section. I was once a medical student myself, so I know that many (if not all) of you will want to jump around this workbook, find the highlights, and try to figure out the reasons why I'm "wrong." You'll then likely attempt to knock your statement out in a single weekend, only to find yourself in a panic on Monday when you're not even half done. This is why it's important that you trust me and trust the process. Fight the impulse to skip ahead, take the time to truly reflect on your own experiences, and complete this workbook's exercises in the order presented. I urge you to invest the time and effort into making your statement the best it can possibly be.

I will tell you right now: By the end of Chapter 8, you're going to have a statement you'll be proud of. However, you won't start writing your first draft until Chapter 5, because writing about yourself is like painting a room—a good bit of work goes into planning and prep. If you're painting a room, buying the right paint, taping off borders, and laying out drop cloths are all about doing the job thoroughly and to the best of your ability; the prep work helps ensure a crisp, clean outcome. When you're writing about yourself, at least the same amount of effort—if not more—is needed for prep.

This workbook is your prep. Some of what you're about to read may seem silly, and some of it may even seem like overkill. You may be right, but I want to give you the tools you need to stand out. If you and another residency applicant are only a hairsbreadth apart in a program director's eyes, I want you to be the one with a knock-it-out-of-the-park statement that gets you the invitation to interview. When you think of skipping a step in this workbook, know that others are not, and these could be the very applicants you'll be competing with. So do your best and do it right: This starts with trusting the process and committing to it.

By the time you're finished, program directors will understand why they should hire *you* over all the other applicants, and you'll be well on your way to Matching in the residency you want.

Let's get started!

# CHAPTER 1

## THE IMPORTANCE OF YOUR STATEMENT

Grades, standardized test scores, research papers, recommendations, clerkships. You've spent your time in med school focused largely on nailing down these crucial important factors, all while trying to learn (and retain) a vast amount of knowledge. You've been trained for years to focus on your numbers, stats, and rankings above all else, and it may be difficult for you to envision how an essay about yourself can affect your residency application.

While your stats *do* matter (and they matter a lot), this doesn't mean it's okay to neglect your personal statement. Far from it. It's natural to feel as if your essay is unimportant, even out-of-place, when compared to other ERAS application elements. However, if you cling to this view too tightly, you're assuming a perilous perspective. Let's examine why.

### UNDERSTANDING THE WEIGHT OF YOUR STATEMENT

I'm sure you've asked yourself if your personal statement is *really* that important. Let me answer that question right now, briefly and concisely, because the answer is a resounding YES.

According to the 2018 NRMP Survey of Program Directors,[1] directors consider almost *three dozen* factors when deciding which applicants to interview, and the personal statement ranks fifth out of the top ten. Take a look for yourself:

---

1 The 2018 NRMP Survey of Program Directors can be found by visiting <https://www.nrmp.org/wp-content/uploads/2018/07/NRMP-2018-Program-Director-Survey-for-WWW.pdf>.

1. USMLE Step 1/COMLEX Level 1 score
2. Letters of recommendation in the specialty
3. Medical Student Performance Evaluation (MSPE/Dean's Letter)
4. USMLE Step 2 CK/COMLEX Level 2 CE score
5. **Personal Statement**
6. Grades in required clerkships
7. Any failed attempt in USMLE/COMLEX
8. Class ranking/quartile
9. Perceived commitment to specialty
10. Personal prior knowledge of the applicant

While the personal statement doesn't rank at the pinnacle of the top-ten factors, it's not at the bottom, either. Even though it will never be quite as important as your USMLE scores, recommendations, and dean's letter, it may surprise you to learn that your statement is *more important* than both your grades in required clerkships and your class ranking.

Why is the statement important enough to rank fifth out of dozens of criteria? It's because, arguably, your essay is the only *subjective* component of your application package. (Even a seemingly subjective letter of recommendation can be reduced to an objective positive or negative.) This means your essay is your one opportunity during the application process to connect with program directors in a personal, *human* way.

Because your statement is subjective, it's also your opportunity to speak to the "soft" criteria that directors cite as meaningful but that are little reflected elsewhere in your application. (These criteria include: perceived commitment to your specialty; leadership qualities; and perceived interest in the specific residency program you've applied to.) The chance to address these areas is no small thing. A score on a standardized test may reflect your knowledge base, but it can't ever offer insight about your level of commitment to your profession.

As a prospective resident headed toward Match Day, it's crucial that you shift your mindset. The Match will be the first time, professionally speaking, that you'll be reaching beyond the fishbowl of your current institution; your world is about to get much, much bigger. From now on, you must assume that you'll be competing with the top ten percent of students from every med school on the planet—because you very well could be.

The most important thing to remember in your new mindset is that other applicants will have scores and recs just as good—if not better than—yours. Therefore, you should view your statement as an unparalleled opportunity: it's the one part of your ERAS package that helps program directors envision who *you* are, and your essay may very well tip the scales in your favor.

Let's review some of the key reasons that you need a memorable statement.

## STANDING OUT IN A SEA OF CANDIDATES

Picture this: you've submitted your full ERAS package to every available residency at your first- and second-choice Match institutions, and you're receiving some initial interest. But even if the director of a particular program pegs you as a top-five candidate, you're still going to be up against others who look just as good by numbers alone as you do. What's going to give you the edge you need to pull ahead of the pack?

When directors are considering neck-and-neck applications, they must begin looking for qualities that distinguish one candidate from another. This is where your personal statement becomes invaluable: a well-written essay will showcase why *you and you alone* are the right candidate for the job. It will display the singular combination of strengths and talents that you can bring to a residency program. It can be the one differentiating factor that leads to an interview!

You're unique and special. You absolutely have experiences and personal convictions that won't show up in your test scores and recs, so you need to approach the essay portion of your application accordingly. You must view your statement as an opportunity, and you should be *excited* about this opportunity: nowhere else can you express what makes you outstanding—both as a physician and as a person.

## FLESHING OUT YOUR QUALIFICATIONS

From the other parts of your ERAS application, any program director will likely be able to glean your goals in your preferred area of medicine. But because your personal statement is subjective, you now have the chance to elaborate on your qualifications in your own words. No other part of your package can explain the spark that's led you to your specialization; no other part can give voice to any distinctive or unusual qualities you have.

Imagine a graduating med student who is applying for a residency in pediatrics. Her numbers and recs are glowing, which is a great starting point. Yet these won't highlight a defining experience she had during a clerkship. They won't pinpoint any of her insights into caring for children, and they certainly won't stress the reason she wants to specialize in children's health. Examples like these are all meaningful, foundational aspects of any prospective resident's profile, ones that can only be expressed in the essay portion of the application.

You have many qualities and qualifications that will make you a wonderful doctor—otherwise you wouldn't have made it this far in the first place. In your essay, you won't need to go into deep detail about every facet of yourself that your numbers can't convey, but you should feature personal attributes that you believe make you the best-qualified candidate for the job.

Remember, too, that not every meaningful qualification is directly related to medicine—in fact, some of the most impressive I've read about have come from well outside the field. For example, if you consider persistence to be a particular strength of yours, an anecdote about overcoming a physical challenge (rather than an academic challenge) could illustrate this perfectly, even though it has nothing at all to do with medicine. As long as you're relating a given quality to the job you want, you shouldn't be afraid to get a little creative. After all, in essay writing, creative usually equals memorable.

## SHOWING YOUR PERSONALITY

Anybody who's ever worked for a living knows that colleagues and co-workers can make-or-break any employment environment. When we're lucky enough to work with people we like and respect, our job becomes easier and much more pleasant. When we work with irritating people who elicit little respect, even a position that looks great on paper can feel like pure drudgery.

You don't ever want others to perceive you as the latter example, even unintentionally. You should use your personal statement to articulate who you are as a professional and *as a prospective colleague*. Let your best nature shine through your writing. USMLE scores don't have a personality, they're just numbers. Your grades are just letters, boring and sterile. These elements are important, of course, but they don't tell program directors anything about what it will be like working with you day in and day out. If you're a cautious optimist, show that in your writing. If you're a "night owl" who'd be at home working the overnight shift, show that. You never know which of your traits will fit in perfectly with the needs of a given program.

Personal statements can be funny, quirky, moving, serious, somber, passionate. Your overall focus should be on landing a face-to-face interview, but you get to decide which parts of your personality to show off. By the time a director finishes reading your essay, she should feel you're an interesting person who would be rewarding to work with. You have a lot to offer any program, so don't hold back!

Hopefully, you now have a better understanding of how important your personal statement truly is. If any of the information I've touched on so far sounds intimidating, don't worry. My method is simple and fairly painless. You don't even need to be a strong writer. All you need is the willingness to work through the steps and follow my lead.

Before we get to the writing process, I'm going to explain the basic requirements for personal statements so you know what the parameters are, and I'll touch on some helpful dos and don'ts. I did promise you step-by-step writing exercises, and we'll get to those soon, but first I'm going to lay out some foundational info in the next chapter.

# CHAPTER 2

## GENERAL GUIDELINES FOR YOUR STATEMENT

Aside from figuring out the actual content of your personal statement (We'll talk about content creation a little bit later), you probably have many questions about what's expected from, and even required for, your essay. That's natural, and it's actually a very good thing—you're already engaged, on some level, in the process of bringing your statement together. "What formatting should I use?" "How long should my statement be?" "How much time should I allot for writing?" are some of the most common before-getting-started questions I've encountered. It's important to know the answers *before* you begin thinking about the content of your statement.

There are a few general guidelines—some essential and some traditional—you'll need to follow, because hewing to them closely will shape your content while also saving you a few headaches. Trying to reinvent the wheel will certainly do more harm than good, so let's review some specs.

### THE MyERAS WEB PORTAL: REQUIREMENTS AND TIPS

Some of the basic requirements for your personal statement come from MyERAS, which is the online portal you'll use to submit your applications. While there are various requirements for each part of your package, there are only two parameters for your statement. They're important parameters, though, and you should know what they are before you put pen to paper.

- A maximum of 28,000 characters. Characters are words, spaces, punctuation marks, and symbols. In sum, 28,000 characters is roughly about 8 pages of single-spaced, 10-point-font text.

- ASCII formatting: When you upload your statement, the text is automatically converted to ASCII encoding. All bolding, underlining, italicizing, or other "fancy" formatting elements are stripped away, so don't plan to use these in your writing in the first place.

While these parameters may look overly simple, they do a lot in terms of framing your essay and giving it structure. However, in my experience, one parameter is much too lax, while the other is very, very helpful. Let's explore each.

Initially, the twenty-eight-hundred character-cap (about forty-six hundred words) might not seem like an impediment—you can certainly say all you need to say in eight pages! However, in my opinion (and I'll be so bold as to say in everyone's opinion), eight pages of text is way too long. This is not a moment when "more" equals "better." A shorter, well-written statement will always be an easier and more remarkable read than one that goes on for pages and pages. You're writing a personal essay; not an autobiography.

You must remember that program directors read dozens, possibly hundreds, of statements when deciding who to invite for an interview. In order to stand out, you need to pen a compelling essay that doesn't mire them in unnecessary details. In terms of length, my best advice is to aim for seven-hundred to eight-hundred words. That's roughly a page and a half of single-spaced text. Stay within this range and you'll be that much more likely to hold any director's attention. If you choose your words carefully, you can make a bigger impression with less text than you could if you used every character available to you.

Conversely, while ASCII may seem limiting, I believe its bare-bones formatting can help you write a stronger statement. Most style guides will tell you that bolding, italics, underlining, and related, should be used sparingly—otherwise writers tend to over-rely on these elements, which is a classic "writing trap," and can make your writing seem lazy. ASCII encoding is actually a gift in disguise; you're obligated to use precise language and carefully crafted words to make a strong impression.

## COMMON PITFALLS

Many personal statements share "big picture" problems. These pitfalls can trip you up if you're not aware of them, so I'll take a moment here to review a few of the most common I've seen. This way you'll know what to avoid right from the top; with this knowledge, you'll be able to lay out a clearer, more original direction for your essay.

The writing process always begins well before any writing actually occurs. You probably know this from years of research papers and clinical studies, but it's worth mentioning here. For the moment, you should be thinking about your statement in broad, more general, proto-writing terms. Here are a few things to keep in mind.

- Always remember that you're applying for a job. It's not appropriate to rehash the essay you wrote to get into med school; very soon, you won't be a student anymore, and you've grown personally and professionally in the last few years.

- Your statement must be personal, but it should also be part sales promo. You want to tell your readers about yourself, yes, but you're also pitching yourself and your skills.

- Write your own statement—don't ask your "writer friend" to do it, and certainly don't pay someone else to do it. Program directors want to know about you in your own unique voice.

- Your statement is an essay, and therefore it must be framed within an essay's standard, fixed structure: a strong introduction, a solid and concise body, and a memorable conclusion. In other words, don't play games with the fundamental structure of an essay. Likewise, writing a poem, song, or play instead isn't going to win you brownie points; it's going to get your application chucked into the rejection pile.

- Avoid using unnecessary medical jargon. Program directors won't be impressed by big words—they already know the lingo, and they almost certainly know it better than you. Jargon is notoriously tricky language, too, and misuse is common. You could easily get into the weeds if you try to show off, so don't do it.

- Don't frame your statement around your own "mystery diagnosis." As personal as your story can feel, this is an old and overused trope. Beyond that, you could create an unconscious bias on the part of the reader. Case in point, a story about your idiopathic rash that turned out to be psychosomatic might lead a director to subconsciously believe you have ongoing/untreated mental health issues. To intentionally deny you an interview because of mental illness would be a violation of the Americans with Disabilities Act, but if a director does this subconsciously, what recourse would you have?

- While your statement must describe you, you must also take pains not to sound too self-centered. (This can be a tough balance to achieve, which is why I'll give you more specific tips on this later.) Be honest and sincere.

- Never use somebody else's writing without permission and/or citations. You probably already know this, but plagiarism is a sure-fire way to take yourself out of the running and ruin your reputation.

My final and maybe most important piece of general advice is not to waste any time explaining why you went into medicine. That's water under the bridge at this point. Instead, focus on the specialty you're concentrating on (and, if applicable, the specific residency program you're applying to). This will evidence your having taken the time to tailor your essay to the job you want.

It may seem like there are a lot of "don'ts" to take into account before you begin writing. In a way you're right. But consider this: none of these rules tell you what you *can* do with your essay, they only tell you what you *shouldn't* do. None of these should hinder your creativity; in fact, they should free you up to consider all the ways you can make your statement striking and truly personal.

To illustrate the type of creativity you can bring to your statement, let me tell you about one of my favorite essays. I read it over five years ago, and it still sticks out in my mind today.

An aspiring resident, much like yourself, was applying for a Match in emergency medicine. She believed her strongest asset was her ability to keep cool and calm in critical situations, as this is essential for emergency room doctors. Instead of writing about a typical high-stress experience for a med student—cramming for the MCAT, the hell of finals week, or her struggles during her clerkships—she painted a dynamic picture about having worked a busy shift in a diner.

This applicant started her story in the middle of a hectic diner-shift, which immediately drew me in. By harnessing her creativity and choosing a story about waiting tables, she instantly made herself stand out in a pile of otherwise bland applications. She went on to describe the ways in which working as a food server and working in an emergency room are similar: constant and ever-changing demands, multiple customers/patients to attend to, and the necessity of grace under fire were some of the parallels she cited. Because she framed her essay so uniquely, her "skills pitch" was especially strong. I was glad to learn she Matched in her first-choice program.

## TIME MANAGEMENT: PROTECTING YOUR WRITING TIME

Good writing takes time. An essay, article, blog post, or review that takes only ten minutes to read very likely has hours (and hours) of work behind it. Think of the last paper you wrote: how long did it take you to write those six, heavily researched pages?

One of the most common mistakes applicants make is underestimating the time commitment required to write a killer statement. Since I recommend a length of about eight hundred words, you might imagine that you can finish your writing in just a few hours. That's far from the truth—and it's a dangerous thing to believe. In fact, because you'll be using fewer words, it will likely take you extra time to complete your personal statement: when every word counts, you need to choose each one much more carefully.

Any polished piece needs several rounds of drafting, rewriting, and editing before the final version emerges. This is no less true with your statement, which arguably will be more important than any non-technical piece you've ever written. You're going to nail this, but you're also going to need plenty of time.

While the application deadline varies for a few specific specializations, for most aspiring residents, the ERAS package is due in early September. Having your statement completed and ready to go by July is ideal, meaning you'll want to start the process at least two months beforehand. That way, you'll have plenty of time to brainstorm, write a rough draft, walk away from it for a while, then begin rewriting, editing, polishing, proofreading, and tailoring it to perfection. (If you're reading this in August, don't worry, you aren't "behind," per se. You may need to clamber a bit, but you'll do just fine if you follow my method.)

I specifically advise starting in May because your statement is the most labor-intensive part of your application. If you have your essay completed by mid-July, you're freeing up late July through September for gathering the more-technical parts of your package *as well as* allowing plenty of time for your professors to read your essay before writing recommendations.

To meet your deadline, you'll want to carve out dedicated blocks of time for the writing process. This is like reserving study time for an exam, but your writing time should be even more focused. Throughout this workbook, I've estimated the amount of time necessary for each writing exercise. Your individual needs may vary, and that's okay. If you find you need more time than I've mapped out for a particular exercise, don't worry about it. The main thing is to approach your writing time in a systematic, protected, manner.

Schedule at least two writing-appointments weekly, preferably three. These appointments are concrete and immoveable: Keep to them strictly. (Pretend you're meeting with a professor or advisor if it helps you stick to your schedule.) These are "no distraction" appointments: no tablets, TVs, or radios allowed, and you should leave your smartphone in the other room. If you're using your laptop, keep that browser closed or turn off the Wi-Fi altogether. (You may need the Internet later on, but not in the initial phases.) The idea is to create a *protected* zone just for writing. Anything else that needs your attention will have to wait until your writing block is over.

No distractions is a big deal, I get it. But at the core of it, when you take away all non-writing stuff, you'll force yourself to focus on what matters. You may think I'm being a little bit mean, but I'm not. I'm preparing you to write the best statement possible, and I want to be frank about the commitment level needed.

---

That covers my general recommendations and guidelines. In the next chapter, we'll start the process of brainstorming (or pre-writing), and I'll walk you through my tried-and-true brainstorming technique. By the end of the pre-writing phase, you'll know the *exact* topic that's right for *your* personal statement.

# CHAPTER 3

## BRAINSTORMING
### ( PRE-WRITING, PART I )

Your personal statement must be, more than anything else, personal. While this may sound like circular logic, *personal* in this context implies that the success of your essay will rely heavily on harnessing your own individual creativity. The pre-writing stage will help you do just that.

The idea of being creative intimidates many med students. After all, your training is science-based, and your discipline is the human body in all its complexities. If you find the idea of tapping into your creative side daunting, know that you're in good company. The thought of being creative is hard for everyone, including established writers and artists. By making it this far into your med school experience, you've already proven that fear is *not* going to hold you back, and that includes any angst you may have about creative writing.

As cliché as it may sound, everyone is creative in some way, including you. Whether you realize it or not, creativity will play a role in your being a doctor almost as much as anything else. Creativity can help you explain a complicated diagnosis to a patient in everyday, relatable terms. It can help you connect with a sick child. It can even help you formulate a surgical approach through complex anatomy. Just like harnessing your creativity will make you a better doctor, it will make you a better writer, too. In your statement, harnessing your creativity is about mining your own experiences and emotions and then using them to craft your writing.

Perhaps the first thing to keep in mind as you begin brainstorming is that your statement is a creative work. Even though you'll be writing an essay, your statement is, at the heart of it, a story—it's not a thesis, not a treatise on the evolution of Western medicine, not a clinical report. These are analysis-based types of writing, which isn't what you need now. Right now you need creative writing that's sincere, honest, evocative, and singularly distinctive.

At this point in your journey, you've been writing analysis-based works for so long that it may initially be difficult for you to shift gears. This is natural—you'll need to "unlearn" a lot to ace your statement. That's why you should begin pre-writing with a dedicated brainstorming session, one that will help you conceptualize your essay as a personal story.

Brainstorming is about getting your ideas together so you can pick and choose the best. Groups and teams often do this kind of "bouncing ideas around," but there are any number of brainstorming-for-one techniques out there. I've tried a few of these, and the one I've found most effective is an idea cloud. Let's look at how to create one.

## CREATING YOUR IDEA CLOUD

An idea cloud is really just a fancy name for all your ideas, all written down in one place. In this case, you'll be jotting down any and all possible ideas for your personal statement's topic. These ideas will be free-floating, like clouds—they don't have to connect to each other in any meaningful way, and they can be semi-formed in the same way that clouds can be wispy around the edges. You don't even need to use complete sentences. You just need to get all your ideas captured.

As we move deeper into the cloud, you'll begin reducing your initial ideas—and the experiences connected to them—down to your strongest ones. By the end, you'll know your statement's topic!

## STEP 1: SEEDING YOUR CLOUD

Seeding your idea cloud is perhaps the most fun part of brainstorming. This is the time for scribbling, messiness, bullet points, or even doodles if you're a particularly visual thinker. Whatever it takes for you to seed your cloud with ideas.

That said, you do want your idea cloud to be highly focused, and this means concentrating your pre-writing on finding experiences you can use to share a meaningful story with your audience of program directors. For this reason, you should make a list of potential-topics categories as soon as you sit down. (For brainstorming, you should also use a pen and paper—not your tablet or laptop—for reasons you'll see later.) Here are the categories I suggest, although you can certainly add others.

- Awards
- Challenges
- Education
- Embarrassing moments
- Falling short
- Goals accomplished
- Hobbies
- Mentors
- Trips
- Work experiences

Now that you've listed your categories, write down any related experiences that come to you. If something out of left field pops into your head, write it down even if—and especially if—it seems unrelated to medicine. Be open. Suspend all judgement as you gather your ideas, turn off your inner critic. There are no "good" ideas, "bad" ideas, or even "silly" ideas at this point. Right now, all ideas are equally valid. Brainstorming is open and free!

As an example of a gem that could "pop into your head," think of the personal statement I mentioned in the last chapter. The student who wrote it used her experience waiting tables as the focal point of her essay, and I'd wager that connecting a diner to an emergency room was a "lightbulb moment" for her. Which is to say, *all* your ideas matter right now. Even though it might not be obvious at first glance, the first time your neighbor paid you for yard work or your summer job at the National Audubon Society could be the spark of your topic.

For a somewhat-less esoteric approach, let's look at the type of experiences you might write under the "Challenges" category:

- Moving away from your best friend
- Bouncing back after a trauma
- Failing a class
- Missing a diagnosis
- Coping with your parents' divorce
- Summiting a mountain

You can add to this list, of course. A challenge can be anything that you had to overcome, or something that you worked overwhelmingly hard to achieve. Your challenges might be related to medicine, but they definitely don't have to be.

### A NOTE ON YOUR STATEMENT AND RED FLAGS

Before we wrap up this section, let's go back to the categories list for a moment. Maybe you didn't notice, but one of the entries I suggested is "Falling short." This is because there's no such thing as a perfect human being, and it's possible you have a red flag or two on your résumé. (It's okay, we've all been there.)

One approach to red flags is to ignore "falling short" moments and hope program directors won't notice. (Hint: they will.) A better approach—a more tenacious and honest approach—is to use your personal statement as an opportunity to meet your red flags head-on. If you needed to repeat a class in med school, had trouble with one of your clerkships, or scored on the low side on a standardized exam, now is the time to talk about it, because unaddressed red flags may prevent you from getting an interview. You don't need to frame your entire statement around them, but this may be your one opportunity to offer some context for any less-than-perfect marks on your record.

Ideally, you'll be able to subtly weave your red flags into your larger story, which will keep your essay from feeling disjointed. Talk about what you *learned* from the "negative" experience. If you do it well, you can illustrate persistence, fortitude, or other positives. Flip that red flag into a hard-won badge of resilience!

I encourage you to seed your cloud over the course of a few days. Use one writing block for initial thoughts, then put your list away overnight. During your next writing block, read through your ideas and add to them. Do this a third time on a third day if you can. At this stage, don't take anything out—jot any and all ideas down.

---

**EXERCISE**

To create your idea cloud, you'll need at least two thirty-minute writing blocks. With your writing time protected, get started by making the categories-list I've suggested. Feel free to add additional categories if they occur to you. Now seed your cloud: write in your ideas and experiences where appropriate. If there are any red flags on your résumé, include them under the "Falling short" category. (Be honest!)

For your second writing block, return to your lists on another day and add more ideas. If possible, schedule a third block and add even more ideas. Do not—*do not*—cross out any ideas.

## STEP 2: IDENTIFY YOUR STRONGEST IDEAS USING A TRAITS LIST

With step one completed, it's time to begin culling your lists and selecting your very best ideas and experiences—the ones that could become your personal statement's topic.

How do you know which ideas are your very best? While this question may seem overwhelming, the answer is actually simple: your best ideas are those that will appeal most to program directors. To identify these, make a color-coded list of the traits you believe are most relevant to your specialty. Write each trait down with a distinctively colored pen, or mark each with a different colored highlighter. You can add as many traits as you like, but here are some examples to get you started:

- Dedication
- Grit
- Humor
- Leadership
- Resilience

In addition, add to your traits list the ACGME's "Six Pillars of Graduate Medical Education." As dry as they sound, these core competencies are the criteria used nationwide to evaluate all residents. Most directors of residency programs can probably recite these by heart, so give the six pillars their due attention.

- Practice-based learning and improvement
- Patient care and procedural skills
- Systems-based practice
- Medical knowledge
- Interpersonal and communication skills
- Professionalism

Now, read through your idea cloud with your first trait in mind. Each time you encounter an experience that demonstrates a specific trait (leadership, for example,) highlight or underline it according to your color key. If it's helpful, you can create a mini key at the top of your idea-cloud page: yellow for leadership, green for resilience, and so on.

Repeat this exercise with each trait on your list until you've gone through all of them. Use multiple colors on any one experience in your idea-cloud where applicable. Ideas marked with more than one color are a good thing—it means you have an experience or anecdote that reflects more than one of the traits you need to succeed.

Keep an open mind as you work. Try to think outside the box as you're connecting ideas and experiences to traits. For example, while something dramatic like overcoming a childhood illness could show resilience, you could also demonstrate resilience by telling the story of going back to school the day after a mortifyingly embarrassing incident.

This phase is meant to be loose and creative, and not at all rushed. Again, it may be helpful to take an overnight break from brainstorming. Resting during creative endeavors is especially important; sometimes distancing ourselves from the task at hand helps incubate ideas. Try to have some fun connecting your ideas and traits; after all, identifying your finest ideas is a little like getting to pat yourself on the back!

---

**EXERCISE:**

To begin identifying your strongest ideas, you'll need at least one forty-five-minute writing block—preferably two so you can get a good night's sleep in between. Place your idea-cloud and traits-list side by side. With your colored highlighters; mark the experiences in your idea cloud that demonstrate the traits on your list. Be sure to create a color key so you won't get confused as you work.

Once you've finished, the next part of this step is to cull your ideas. Take a new sheet of paper and create colored columns for each of your traits. For those ideas that you've marked with more than one color, put it in every trait column where it applies. Do this slowly; you don't want to miss an extraordinary idea-to-trait connection by going too quickly.

With that done, go ahead and cross out any ideas and experiences that appear in only one column. These are your "only okay" ideas, so it's best to let them go now. Those that appear in three or more columns are your strongest ideas. Circle these, then copy them on a clean sheet of paper. From here on out, we'll be calling this newly created list your *culled-idea-cloud*.

---

**EXERCISE:**

To begin culling your ideas, you'll need one forty-five-minute writing block, preferably two. On a new sheet of paper, create a color-coded column for each trait you've identified and write in every idea/experience that exhibits that trait. Do this slowly. Then cross off any experiences that aren't listed in more than one column and bid goodbye to these. Circle any experiences appearing in three or more columns.

Write the circled ideas on a clean sheet of paper. This is your culled-idea-cloud, and one of the ideas listed here will very probably become your statement's topic.

---

## STEP 3: DESCRIBE YOUR SPECIALTY

You've now merged your idea cloud and your trait list into one culled-idea-cloud, and you've jettisoned your more mediocre ideas in the process. Well done. Now put aside your culled-idea-cloud for the moment. It's time to switch gears and think about the specific language that describes your specialty. Why? Because this more-precise language will give you ideas on shaping your essay to your chosen area of medicine.

Take out a clean sheet of paper and begin brainstorming again. Think of your specialty and write down any descriptive words related to it. (If it helps, close your eyes and picture yourself in practice.) If you have two or three specialty possibilities, do this for each of them.

For example, if you're pursuing a pediatrics residency, descriptive words would be:

- Babies
- Children
- Compassion
- Energy
- Humor
- Parents
- Stickers

Note "Stickers" on the list above. If a word that's far-afield jumps into your head, write it down anyway, even if it seems ridiculous. In this case, I included the word *stickers* because I have a vivid memory of my pediatrician letting me choose my "good behavior" sticker at the end of a checkup. If I were writing an essay, this memory might serve as my launching pad. That's the thing about creativity—you never know where it'll lead you.

As a part of your language-list, you should also write down anything about yourself that you believe gives you an edge in your chosen field. In keeping with the pediatrics example, you might write down that you've memorized hundreds of knock-knock jokes or that you're a fan of *Star Wars*, since these could help you relate to the children who will be your patients.

**EXERCISE:**

For this exercise, you'll need one thirty-minute writing block for each of your specialty possibilities; work through them one at a time. For each specialty, make the language-list I've outlined above. Remain open to all ideas and all words as you work. Let your creativity lead you.

## STEP 4: RELATE YOUR EXPERIENCES TO YOUR SPECIALTY

The next step is to place your culled-idea-cloud and your specialty-language-list side by side on the table in front of you. Study them. Contemplate. Think about how they relate to each other. Relax as you let your mind free-form connections.

Grab a fresh sheet of paper. At the top of the page, write down both your specialty and the words from your language-list. Now draw three columns. In each column, write down one related experience from your culled-idea-cloud. Now write down free-formed connections as they come to you. Leave some space in between each for fleshing out your connections a little. Do this again for each of your other possible specialties.

For example, if your desired specialty is emergency medicine, you might think of a connection that's fairly obvious (like the time you needed to call an ambulance for a loved one), or it can be related in a non-medical way (like the waiting-tables example used earlier in the book). Here are some other examples of free-form connections linked to emergency medicine.

- Babysitting
- Compassion
- Grace under fire
- Time management

When you're ready, start expanding on each connection using bullet points, phrases, or simple words. Don't write sentences during this step. Sentences require grammar, and grammar is one of creativity's strongest buzz kills.

Here's what the list above could become once you start expanding:

- Babysitting
    Diapers and throw-up
    Hectic
    Unsupervised position

- Compassion
    Empathy
    Hand-holding
    Non-judgment

- Grace under Fire
    Daily meditation practice
    Gut instincts
    Leadership

- Time management
    Forced focus
    Sacrificed social life
    Self-discipline

Free-forming is one of creativity's greatest gift—there's no telling what kind of brilliant idea you'll come up with—so remember that there are no incorrect answers here. All you're doing at this point is fleshing out the stuff you've already identified as strong. Let your connections form naturally and organically, and don't question whether or not a particular connection "deserves" to be on your list. You had the idea for a reason. Trust yourself.

For instance, take a look at "Diapers and throw-up" under "Babysitting." Why is this here? It's because emergency room doctors routinely get vomited on, urinated on, coughed on, and they otherwise experience a whole host of messy stuff that most people find gross. If you're comfortable with this very-integral but somewhat-icky part of emergency medicine, you'll likely want to mention it in your personal statement. Likewise, you'll see "Daily meditation practice" listed under "Grace under fire." These two things might not go together in an obvious way, but meditation is an excellent stress-management tool—if it's a part of your daily (or weekly) routine and helps you keep your cool, you can talk about it in your essay.

Take as much time with this stage as you need. As you're free-forming connections, you'll probably find that you have a lot to say about some ideas but not much about others. That's expected, and it's an important part of the process. Oddly enough, at this stage, you're both narrowing down your potential topics, as well as expanding on your strongest ideas. (Creativity works like that—try not to think about the paradox too much or you might get a headache.)

---

**EXERCISE:**
Reserve at least two one-hour writing blocks for this exercise, preferably separated by one night's rest. For each of your potential specialties, put your language-list next to your culled-idea-cloud. Create the template as directed above. Free-form as many connections as you can, expanding on each as needed. Write down all connections as your creativity flows from your pen. Don't rush: add more writing blocks if you need more time.

---

## STEP 5: RANK THE BEST OF THE BEST

Now that you've identified and fleshed out your already-strong ideas, your final step in the brainstorming process is to rank them based on how relevant they are to your desired specialty.

You can use any rating system you like, but I think keeping it simple is best: a good old-fashioned one-to-ten scale will do just fine. The highest scores go to any ideas in your culled-idea-cloud that relate to several key traits on your list AND that were relatively easy for you to flesh out.

After you've ranked your choices, take out a new sheet of paper and create a "best of the best" list. Include any idea or experience that you ranked seven or above. (Go back and look at the "Six Pillars of Graduate Medical Education" in Step 2 if it helps.) You should now have only those stories and experiences that will strongly interest program directors.

Any topic on your "best of the best" list would be fantastic foundational material for a personal statement. However, you're not just looking for a strong idea, you're looking for the idea that excites you, the thing you *want* to write about. In creative writing, passion counts for a lot.

It's okay if a single "best of the best" idea doesn't command your attention right now. You've done a ton of work, and you're probably a bit burned out from brainstorming. It happens. As they say, things will look brighter in the morning.

But before you call it quits for the day, on the reverse side of your "best of the best" page, jot down two or three sentences about the life-lessons you learned from each experience, and how those lessons relate to your chosen specialty. These should be full sentences, but they don't have to be fancy ones—I promise no one needs to see them but you. Essentially, these are notes to yourself; they will be helpful when you begin writing. For example, if you're applying to a physical medicine and rehabilitation residency, you might write something to the effect of, "After tearing my ACL in high school, I knew playing Division I collegiate basketball wasn't in my future. However, in order to become a part of the team I grew up idolizing, I joined the athletic training program, which introduced me to the scope and breadth of physical medicine and rehabilitation. The direction of my life changed forever."

Now it's time for a break. Put your "best of the best" list aside for a few days. Stuff it in a drawer (along with all your other lists and pages) and walk away. Now that you know you'll be working with excellent material, free up your conscious mind for a while. When you open that drawer a few days later, the topic for your statement will jump out at you. This is the idea you're most excited about viscerally; this is the idea you can write the most passionately about. Congratulations!

---

**EXERCISE:**

To rank your choices, set aside one forty-five-minute writing block—plus at least one good night's sleep. For each potential specialty, rank your ideas. Write anything scoring seven or higher on a new "best of the best" list. Flip the page over and write one or two "life lessons" sentences for each idea.

Put the paper away overnight, or preferably for a few days. When you come back to it, one potential topic above all others will speak to you. This is your statement's topic; this is the seed of your first draft.

---

As you might've guessed, we're at the end of the brainstorming phase. We'll delve into your first draft shortly, but before we get into the nitty-gritty of writing, in the next chapter I'm going to share some general tips about effective creative writing. If nothing else, these tips will help steer you away from technical, analytical writing and will put you in a storytelling mindset.

# CHAPTER 4

## CREATIVE WRITING 101
### ( PRE-WRITING, PART II )

Even with your initial pre-writing completed, I expect you're still a little apprehensive about the writing process itself, especially if you don't think of yourself as a strong writer. That's good, that's natural. You're nervous because nailing your personal statement is important to you—if you didn't care, you wouldn't be worried. While the work you've done so far might not seem like much in terms of "real" writing, your efforts truly are the foundation for all that will follow.

Because you've worked diligently through my idea-cloud brainstorming method and systematically selected your topic, the hardest part of the writing process is behind you. You can rest easy, in a sense: you know you'll be working with tremendous material. Now you can start thinking about ways to present your content creatively and compellingly.

Writing creatively and compellingly might sound intimidating, but there's no need to be overly nervous. Writing is merely a form of communication, and I'll wager that you communicate in writing all the time—texts, emails, and social media posts are probably a part of your everyday. While your statement needs to be more formal than an email to your buddy, it doesn't have to be lofty, stuffy, or elevated. Your goal is to let your personality and uniqueness shine; if you let yourself get mired in literary gymnastics, you're not going to sound like you. Crisp, clear language is really all you need.

Keep in mind, too, that although your statement needs to be well-written, it won't be judged as a piece of writing, per se. There's no

English teacher grading your essay, and there's no literary-committee-on-high scouring your text for symbolism or allegory. Rather, your statement is the creative, subjective part of your ERAS package. It needs to do three primary things: communicate why you're right for the job, reflect who you are as an individual, and relay a memorable story. To help you do that, I've written this chapter as a crash course on creative-writing-tips for essays.

Remember, you're not drafting your statement just yet; you're still in the pre-writing stage. The exercises in this section are designed to kickstart your creative-writing juices. As you work through them, try to have a little fun. Work and play are not always mutually exclusive.

## SHOW, DON'T TELL

The first rule of creative writing—from poetry, to songwriting, to novels, to essays—is "Show, don't tell." *Telling* your readers a story is like handing out sleeping pills. *Showing*, on the other hand, invites your readers to come into your story *with* you.

You probably know the saying, "A picture is worth a thousand words." You can't include images in your personal statement, of course, but you can and *must* paint a picture with your words. Ask yourself which is the more powerful of these two examples:

I am a resilient person who has overcome many challenges in my life.

The truck skidded toward me. The next thing I knew, I was in a hospital room. My doctor said I would never walk again, but three years later she greeted me at the finish line of my first half-marathon race.

There's no question that the second example is more poignant and engaging. It *shows* resilience instead of telling the reader that resilience is a quality you have. It invests the reader in your story.

When it comes to showing language, strong verbs are key. The English language is rich; our words have specific meanings and connotations, and verbs in particular are multifaceted. You must use this to your advantage in your writing.

Here's a simple example. If you write, "I walked across the room," you're not doing much to put a picture in the reader's head. You could add an adverb (walked quickly), but that's still not terribly visual. The verb *walked* is flat, almost insipid; instead, try a stronger, more specific verb like *galloped, marched, pranced, scampered,* or *trotted.* These stronger verbs do double-duty; each has its own shade of meaning (which gives the reader an image to hold onto) while also conveying the forward-motion of walking.

Since our language has so many synonyms, I strongly encourage you to make friends with a thesaurus during this second pre-writing phase. Reviewing synonyms creates a fresh cache of words in the mind; you'll be able to easily call on these more-robust words when needed. Using a print thesaurus is ideal, but online versions are okay, too. If you go the digital route, try the online version of Merriam Webster's.

---

**EXERCISE:**

For this exercise, you'll need at least one half-hour writing block. Open up a thesaurus, preferably a print version that you can thumb through freely. (Roget's is a good choice.) Choose a word, then read the synonyms for that word. Do it again. And again. Let your curiosity lead you. Pay attention to the trove of options for any given entry, and jot down any words that particularly resonate with you. Do this for the full half-hour or until you get a "feel" for the richness that synonyms offer. Don't be surprised if you find yourself enjoying the process.

Showing, not telling, also means using vivid, visual language. If your essay were a painting, each distinctive word would be a brush-stroke—each adds color and boldness and zest to your canvas. Weak and bland words contribute nothing to your painting and only mute your palate. Adjectives and adverbs might add a touch of extra pigment to your paint, but they can only boost your writing by so much before wordiness takes over; unfortunately, wordiness has the same effect as using a sepia filter on even the most vivid of images.

Because visual language is notoriously hard to describe, we'll jump right into an example that shows (rather than tells) you what I mean. The first paragraph below is deliberately bland. The second shows the power of visual language.

> I was climbing a cliff overlooking San Francisco Bay. My water bottle had just fallen more than two-hundred feet. My heart pounded, and my arms shook.

> The indigo water of San Francisco Bay lay two-hundred feet below me, sparkling in the late afternoon sun. My heart pounding, I watched in shock as my water bottle plummeted down the cliff. My arms quivered as I struggled to pull myself a few inches higher.

The second example puts the reader in the scene, looking at the dark blue ocean below and watching the water bottle plunge into the bay. It's gripping and dramatic. "My arms quivered" paired with the verb "struggled" creates a fantastic image and adds a tension that's absent from the first example almost entirely.

To transform the first paragraph into the second one, I did two main things. First, I packed in five descriptive visual-language verbs (*sparkling, pounding, plummeted, quivered, struggled*), and I also created an immersive perspective for the reader. While I wrote both paragraphs in the first-person (that is, using *I* instead of *you* [second person] or *s/he*, [third person]), the latter paragraph employs what's called a close first-person: I wrote as if the scene were taking place in the *here and now*, rather than as a personal experience that happened in the past. Employing the close first-person is an excellent way of hooking your readers.

If you want to explore close first-person perspectives further, pick up your favorite twenty-first-century novel—any one where the main character speaks primarily in *I*—and bring a reviewer's eye to it. Is there any distance between the protagonist and the author who wrote her? The answer is usually no: the author and the protagonist read as one and the same person. Your essay isn't fiction, but you are in fact both the author of your story and the protagonist in it. Don't talk about what you did, *describe* it as if the action were taking place right now.

As for the five showing verbs I used: if you'd like some further visual-language examples, try reading the screenplay of your favorite movie. Excluding dialogue, screenwriters are mostly restricted to what they can show, so they rely on succinct yet powerful descriptions as they build a world for each story. It's worth noting though, that screenwriting has highly specific conventions: to allow screenwriters to focus on descriptive writing, grammar, flow, and other structural elements of English largely get thrown out the window. In this sense, don't write like a screenwriter in your essay.

Visual writing and close first-person use are important, but there's another indispensable component to showing not telling: reader engagement. Many of the statements I've read don't leave room for the reader to draw conclusions, which risks boring the audience to death. I understand the tendency to over-expound—as a med student, you've been trained in explaining. From outlining the circulatory system to discussing a multifaceted diagnosis, your days have been full of explanations. In creative writing, however, you don't need to explain, you need to *engage*. As I said, writing is a form of communication, and communication is a two-way street; engaging readers creates a conversation-in-writing of sorts. Readers will draw conclusions and understand your message if your work is clear and compelling. As proof, let's go back to the last example for a moment.

> The indigo water of San Francisco Bay lay two-hundred feet below me, sparkling in the late afternoon sun. My heart pounding, I watched in shock as my water bottle plummeted down the cliff. My arms quivered as I struggled to pull myself a few inches higher.

Where in this example does it say the author is rock climbing? Nowhere! Yet readers immediately understand that this scene is about scaling a bluff. Why? Because the author used descriptive, visual, close-first-person language. Everything readers need to know about the "what and where" of the scene is embedded in the words themselves.

---

**EXERCISE:**

Set aside a minimum of two thirty-minute writing blocks or one sixty-minute block. (Unlike previous exercises, you don't need to plan resting time in between, although you can take a break midway if you want.) The first part of your very onerous task is to spend at least a half-hour online reading the screenplay for your favorite movie. (A good place to start is the Internet Movie Script Database [IMSDb].) As you're reading, ignore the grammar, skim through the dialog. Focus on the descriptive language used for each scene. Watch as the screenwriter crafts a picture in each.

For the remaining thirty minutes, your task is even more torturous: go read your favorite contemporary first-person novel. Just about any chapter will do, but do avoid the first chapter for this exercise, as this is often where somewhat-heavy exposition (i.e. explaining) lives, and that's not what you need to focus on now. Pay attention to how close the first-person perspective is, even if the novel itself is framed in the past. How immediate, how engaging, does the first-person feel?

## STORYTELLING WITHIN AN ESSAY FORMAT

It's crucial to your mindset to remember that you're crafting a story in your essay. This means using a storytelling structure is a must. It will help you draw readers in, hold their attention until the end, and express your message in your own voice.

At the same time, your personal statement is first and foremost an essay, and so it *must* have an essay's *fixed* structure: an introduction, a body, and a conclusion—and these elements must be employed in this order. I briefly mentioned this fixed structure in Chapter 2, but it's worth restating here because, by contrast, story-structures are much less rigid; every story must have a beginning, a middle, and an end, but not necessarily in that order. This means the beginning-middle-end in storytelling works differently from the introduction-body-conclusion of an essay. It's up to you to meld these two very different formats effectively (The middle of your story, for example, could also be the introduction of your essay.), and I'm going to help you do just that.

Stories offer you structure-options that essays simply don't, and this means you get to decide where your tale opens. Your story can be chronological, but you can also start in the middle before circling back to the beginning and then later filling in the ending. You can also open at the ending, then go back and address the beginning and the middle (almost like a flashback). Whichever option you choose, your story should take readers on a journey. Let's take a look at each story-structure option a bit further.

**Chronological:** This is when you begin at the beginning and continue your story straight through to the end. It's the simplest of story structures, but it has the considerable benefits of clarity, straightforwardness, and ease of reading.

***En medias res:*** This is a Latin term we've borrowed. It translates literally to "in the middle of things." With this technique, you open smack in the middle of the action, just like in the San Francisco Bay example. *En medias res* has perhaps the greatest potential for pulling a reader in, but if you use it, you must be careful to fully establish your beginning, while also finding a way to transition smoothly to your ending.

**Ending first:** This is a less conventional choice, but it can work in some cases. This is when you start with your story's climax ("I summoned one last burst of energy and surged over the finish line, winning the race.") and then address the other parts. Ending-first is a little risky for various reasons, especially because you'll have work a little harder to restate the climax in an impactful, but fresh, way as you conclude your essay. There's also some grammar trip-ups here: there's this terrible thing in English called the past-perfect tense, and if you're starting at the end, you'll need to use this tense properly while still creating an immersive experience for your readers. If you don't know what the past-perfect tense is, don't choose this option.

When we combine a story's flexible beginning-middle-end with an essay's fixed intro-body-conclusion, we get pieces that look like this:

**Introduction:** The intro of your essay must immediately capture your readers' attention and invite them into your story, while *also* containing the thesis statement of your essay (i.e., you're the best candidate for the residency). Your intro needs to do this whether you're starting your story at the beginning, middle, or end.

**Body:** The body of your essay must expand on and support your thesis statement, while also keeping your story's momentum going. Though you'll be using less than eight-hundred words, it can still be challenging to avoid "mid-essay sag," in your first draft, but don't worry. (Later on, you'll begin editing. This is when you'll be cutting things down and streamlining.) The body of your essay is also where your story gets wrapped up—only very rarely will a story's ending make its way into an essay's conclusion. Lastly, the body must do one other thing as well: offer you a natural flow into your concluding paragraph.

**Conclusion:** Here is where you explicitly relate your story's content to your essay's thesis, while also restating that thesis in a fresh new way; the two come together as you finish things up. Something like, "My year as an US Army medic offered me the hands-on skills used in field medicine . . ." might be an appropriate start to a conclusion if you're applying to a residency at a rural hospital.

Give some thought to what story-structure approach will be most effective for the topic you've chosen. If the idea of playing with the story-structure feels scary at all, remember that tons of amazing statements have been written in simple chronological order. Yours can be too.

---

**EXERCISE:**
Set aside at least one forty-five-minute writing block. Keeping in mind the differences between essay-structure and story-structure, begin thinking about the overall presentation of your statement. Play with storytelling's flexible structure as you sketch out a few broad, loose outlines for your statement—your outlines must follow an essay's fixed structure and must include a beginning, middle, and an end for your story. Don't overthink it, but do try to pull together some structure options for your first draft.

## STRIKING THE RIGHT TONE

The tone in creative writing (in any writing, really) conveys a lot, and in the case of your essay, you want your tone to reflect who you are as a person *and* as a professional. You probably think of "professional" as meaning "formal and straight-laced," but that's a narrow and somewhat dated view; clarity and sincerity count for much more than you likely expect. I told you earlier that your personal statement doesn't need to be lofty or stuffy, and I stand by that. Unless you yourself are the lofty, stuffy sort, don't strive for five-dollar words and long, winding sentences. Instead, choose a tone that allows lots of room for your personality to show through.

The tone I am using in this book is conversational, even though as a doctor and former academic physician, I could've gone for a formal, technical (and dry as dirt) tone. Instead, I'm writing as if I were speaking directly to you, the reader; this establishes a rapport between us and also offers a glimpse of who I am because my personality is naturally embedded in the text itself. My advice is that you adopt a similar conversational tone in your statement: it'll keep you comfortable in your own skin as you write.

Be careful, though, because there *is* a difference between conversational and casual. While it's true that I'm writing to you conversationally, I'm also writing professionally: my text is relatable, well-organized, mechanically sound, and it states my points clearly. (Or at least that's what my editor tells me). In your essay, you will need to be equally mindful of proper grammar, spelling, and organization. Even when written conversationally, your statement is still a professional document, not a casual one. It's not a text message to your friend or an email to your dad: you're applying for a job.

However, within the framework of professionally conversational, you do have a lot of freedom. For example, you can pick an underlying tone that's also:

- Dramatic
- Inspirational
- Playful
- Quirky
- Witty

Above all, the tone you choose should underscore your "you-ness"—you don't want to do something like adopting humorous tone when you're not a humorous person. If you do, your writing will come out stilted, forced, and probably dry. Worse still, if you do manage to score a couple of interviews, program directors won't be meeting the person they were expecting, which could cost you your residency slot.

How do you know which underlying tone is best for you? It's not a question with a straightforward answer, but you can sleuth around for some clues. For one thing, ask a few of your friends to describe your personality in five adjectives. If a quality comes up often, this says a lot about how you relate to others. Another trick is to record yourself as you're telling a story to someone you know well—any story will do, even if you're just talking about something that happened at the grocery store. As you play back the recording, listen to the words you chose, the cadence of your voice, and the syllables or words you naturally emphasize. That's what your statement's tone should sound like, spruced up a bit for professional presentation.

---

**EXERCISE:**

For the next forty-five minutes, free-write a conversational-style paragraph or two on the topic of your choosing. Don't worry about grammar and spelling and professionalism just yet—simply get one- to two-hundred words down. When you're finished, read the paragraph(s) aloud a few times. Can you hear a natural underlying tone emerge? That's the basis of what "you" sound like in writing.

## BUILDING A PERSONAL BRAND

Building a personal brand isn't something that you'll find in most creative-writing advice, but it's applicable in this instance. While branding might seem strange in relation to applying for a residency, it shouldn't; the two converge in an important way.

In the world of advertising and marketing, a company's brand is more than just its logo. Branding represents a company's identity as a whole—who they are and what they do, the value they provide, their customer service, and much more.

A company's brand influences the way consumers think of them. For example, Apple's brand is about lifestyle, freedom, and innovation, all combined with a signature "hipness" factor. Alternately, Google's brand is about accessibility, utility, and quality, all of which is tinged with a distinct, progressive quirkiness. With Apple and Google being two of the most successful companies in the world, they're doing something right with their branding!

Because it's still so early in your career, you don't have a brand yet. That's okay, but you should begin thinking of one as you craft your essay. At this point, your brand is the answer to the question, "What kind of doctor will I be?" The other parts of your application will offer hard facts and stats, but your brand is about your *identity*. In your essay, you want to speak about your competency and drive as an emerging doctor of course, but you also want to highlight the qualities (including your personality) that you want others to think of when they think of you. An obstetrician might want a brand that's warm and nurturing, while a cardiac surgeon would more likely want a brand that emphasizes steady hands and cool headedness.

In the last chapter, you created a list of traits related to the specialty you want. (See Chapter 3, Step 2.) Out of all the work you've done so far, these traits will help you decide on the overarching elements of your emerging personal brand. Once you've identified this, it will inform much about your statement, from the underlying tone to the language you use.

> **EXERCISE:**
> For this exercise, reserve two thirty-minute writing blocks, preferably with at least a few hours in between. Pull out all the lists you made in Chapter 3. While giving some extra consideration to your traits list, review your lists with an eye for building a personal brand. Comb through them. An image of who you are as an emerging doctor will begin to form. Make any notes on a clean sheet of paper so you can keep them next to you when you begin drafting your statement.

Creative writing is a subject I could delve into much more deeply, but it's not necessary. I've outlined the biggest tips you need; keep these in mind as you move forward. Coming up next, I'll walk you through the process of writing your first draft.

# CHAPTER 5

## WRITING YOUR FIRST DRAFT

It's time to start writing your first draft. I know this can seem scary, but I want you to stay positive and keep an open mind, because you're more prepared than you probably think. You've already done a lot of work: you've picked out the topic for your personal statement, and you have a whole trove of lists, ideas, notes, and writing snippets to call on if you get stuck. You know the structure your essay needs to take, you've thought about how you want to present your story within that structure, and you know the tone you'll be writing in. You're way ahead of the game already!

Even with all the work you've done so far, writing your first draft still might feel intimidating. Don't worry. Here's the big secret about first drafts: They stink. All of them. There's this myth out there that writing flows magically from an author's fingertips until a whole and perfect piece pops out. Nothing could be further from the truth. By the time any text is ready to be sent out into the larger world, the author has spent a whole lot of time drafting, revising, rewriting, editing, and proofreading. It's all a part of the writing process, and it all starts with a first draft.

Since you're about to write your first draft, now's a good time to define what, exactly, a draft is. According to Merriam Webster's, a draft is "a preliminary sketch, outline, or version." A draft, then, isn't supposed to be finished or polished. It's an inherently imperfect thing. There'll be plenty of time to worry about refinements later, but for the time being, imperfect is what you're going for. So take a deep breath and let yourself off the "excellence" hook just this once.

I've known too many med students who've weighed themselves down with unrealistic first-draft expectations; all this does is create a lot of frustration that ultimately slows the writing process down. For your first draft, your goal is simply to get a whole statement written without stressing about "bad" writing. In fact, many authors will tell you that a "bad" first draft is a *necessary* step on the path to crafting something spectacular.

For this chapter, I recommend reading it fully through once, then sitting down to write. As you write, refer back to the pointers here as needed.

## USING THE ACTIVE VOICE

As you're writing your personal statement, you'll need to stay in the active voice throughout. In the last chapter, we talked about the tone of your essay—you're going for conversational, with an underlying tone (quirky, inspirational, etc.) of your choosing. An important tool in setting that tone is the active voice.

There are two main various voices in English: the active voice and the passive voice. A lot can be said about each, but we don't need to get into detail here. What you do need to know is that the active voice makes your writing clear and alive, while its "opposite," the passive voice, makes you sound like an eighteenth-century relic. Can you guess which one will land you a residency interview?

As a quick refresher, the active voice means that the subject of your sentence *acts* on the object of the verb—as in, "I climbed the mountain." In the passive voice, the object of the verb is the sentence's subject, and the action is *passed onto it*—as in, "The mountain was climbed by me." Since this is a workbook and not a grammar, I've simplified this explanation somewhat, but suffice to say, invigorate your story—and your essay as a whole—by staying primarily in the active voice.

I'm mentioning active and passive voices right off the bat because many scientific and medical texts still use the passive voice often—

industry convention requires it. You've probably read medical texts written primarily in the passive voice a thousand times, and because passive language has an elevated feel to it, you may make the mistake of trying to emulate it in your writing. Please don't.

In your essay, the only time to frame a sentence in the passive voice is if you're deliberately trying not to blame one person or entity for something that's gone wrong. Because the passive voice doesn't focus on the actor in a sentence, that actor can be omitted entirely. In the active voice, the sentence "My team leader missed the diagnosis, and we were in a panic," clearly places the blame on the team leader (who, in this example, is the actor.) In the passive voice, you can leave out the actor altogether. "The diagnosis was missed, and we were in a panic." In this passive-construction sentence, no one person gets the blame, yet it still sounds professional and polished. (If you've ever wondered why "Mistakes were made," is a favorite of politicians, now you know.)

Other than this one exception, there's very little room for the passive voice in your statement. You'll have to trust me on this one— stay in the active voice.

## STRENGTHENING YOUR FOCUS

We've already talked about the myriad things your personal statement must achieve, and in the midst of all that, it can be easy to lose sight of the reason you're writing your essay in the first place: to get a job. While you don't need to talk excessively about your specialty or the specific residency program you're applying to, these considerations should be at the fore of your mind's eye as you work; they're overarching themes that will color all you write.

I encourage you to physically write a note to yourself at the top of your first draft. Something as simple as, "Statement for pediatrics residency" will keep you grounded and thinking about your goal as you work. Alternatively, you could tack an index card over your desk or put a sticky note near your keyboard. Whatever method you choose, the idea is literally not to lose sight of what you're doing. When you see your purpose every time you look up, you'll be able to hone in on your goal that much more intensely.

Likewise you should have all the notes, lists, and writing snippets you've created so far close at hand so you can refer back to them as needed. I advise having them fanned out on your desk as you work, but if this isn't possible, at least have them in a stack within arm's reach. All the work you've already done is going into your essay in one form or another, even if only conceptually. Straining to remember an idea you've already had or grasping for a word you've already identified as strong will only slow down your writing and frustrate you. You want your first-draft process to be as smooth as possible, and smooth largely means focused. Let the work you've already done be your inspiration.

## PUTTING PEN TO PAPER

Putting pen to paper after all this work should be an exciting prospect! My advice is to write your first draft in one sitting, and to do so as quickly as possible. Schedule a ninety-minute writing block and commit to working non-stop until you have a full essay. This might sound overwhelming but writing eight-hundred words in ninety minutes works out to less than ten words a minute. (You can do that, no sweat!) This ninety-minute block allows for thinking time as well, so your pace won't feel rushed even though you'll be writing fairly quick.

### A NOTE ON WRITING AN OUTLINE

Sometime during your academic career, someone probably stressed the importance of creating a detailed outline before you begin writing. If you've found outlines helpful in the past, go ahead and sketch one now—something more formal and comprehensive than the outlines you created in Chapter 4. An outline isn't mandatory, though; some writers find freewriting during the first-draft stage to be a more creative approach. Do whichever works best for you.

It's important that you write your first draft without letting your inner critic get in your way—your personal statement is going to be incredible by the time you're done, so banish that negativity. Even if you don't know how to spell a word or find yourself unsure of a comma placement, don't stop; keep moving forward. No one is going to see your first draft but you, and at this point, there's no one keeping score of your mistakes. The first draft is about getting content onto the page; you can fix things up at other points in the process. In other words, write now, worry later.

In fact, you shouldn't even be concerned right now about keeping to your word count. Once you've hit your "writing flow," let the words come as they may. You can always tighten your language later, so if your first draft comes to say, twelve-hundred words (That's a whopping pace of thirteen words per ninety-minute writing block), that's perfectly fine. Also, for the time being, don't concern yourself too much with precise word choice. You did some good work with a thesaurus in the last chapter, and you'll return to it in the next chapter. For now, if you find yourself employing a bunch of bland verbs, or if you notice you've written the word *amazing* ten times, leave it be.

Many writers also need to repeat a lot in order to get the thoughts in their head onto the page. This is very common and totally okay at this point. While you don't want to repeat any more than is absolutely necessary in your final version, you're not concerned with your final version right now. (It will become easier to identify instances of repeating later on, anyhow.) If you need to write a phrase like, "I'm interested in this specialty because . . ." five times in order to state five different reasons for your interest, go ahead. Do whatever you need to do to get your thoughts out of your head and into your essay.

As you're drafting your introduction and body, you should also be thinking ahead to the conclusion. Sometimes, the act of writing itself will birth a strong conclusion, but more often, it's helpful to have a loose idea of how you want to wrap your essay up. (Either way, you'll probably draft several iterations of your conclusion before you're happy with it). Just remember that your conclusion must tie into your thesis (i.e., "I'm right for this job"). How you transition from the body of your essay to that conclusion is up to you.

## BREAKING CONVENTION IN CASE OF EMERGENCY

Writing doesn't come easily to most of us. That's okay, everyone has their own talents, and everyone has an area or two where they don't shine quite as brightly. If you find yourself really struggling as you try to write, if you've sat through at least two ninety-minute writing blocks but the words simply won't come, if you're undeniably in the throes of a writing emergency, you can try using text-to-speech software instead. Sit down and narrate your story conversationally as if you were speaking to a grandparent, aunt, or mentor. (In other words, pretend you're talking to someone who knows you well, and to whom you always speak respectfully.) Don't worry about your formal intro or conclusion for the moment. Just get your story out; you can write in the necessary structural elements of an essay later.

A word of caution: only employ text-to-speech software after an honest effort, because there are nuanced differences between speaking and writing. If you do go this route, you must be prepared to do a good amount of extra work in the rewriting and editing phases. However, if your writer's block feels truly insurmountable, text-to-speech can help you get a very rough, audio-based-draft together. From here, you'll be on your way to writing your first draft!

### EXERCISE

Gather together all your notes, psych yourself up, and sit yourself down at your desk. Commit to a ninety-minute writing block; "protected writing time" is especially crucial for this exercise, so take extra pains to ensure a distraction-free environment.

Begin writing your first draft, and write until you have a whole essay from intro to conclusion. Remember to use the active voice, but also make sure you turn off your inner critic. For now, don't worry about your mistakes, don't worry about "bad" writing. Give your full attention to crafting your story and creating your essay. When you have a whole first draft, stop writing.

The last step in the first-draft process may be a surprising one: walk away. Even if you're on a roll, resist the urge to edit, resist the urge to rewrite. Let your words and work rest for a while. For a few days, forget about your personal statement entirely. Go do something fun (Yes, really!) and relax. Your draft will be ready for you when you're ready for it.

---

Well done. You now have a first draft! No matter how rough your draft is, you've achieved a milestone, and things can only get better from here. In the next chapter, I'll talk about the importance of editing and rewriting, and I'll give you some tips on how to edit your personal statement effectively and efficiently.

# CHAPTER 6

## YOUR SECOND AND THIRD DRAFTS
### ( EDITING, PART I )

"Every first draft is perfect because all the first draft has to do is exist." This quote, usually attributed to novelist Jane Smiley, holds words of wisdom. Now that you've written your first draft, you have a perfectly imperfect gem to work with. From here, you're going to take that gem, shape it, remove any flaws, sand it, and polish it. Before long, you'll have a stunning jewel reflecting your very best.

Good writing is rewriting. No writer gets it perfect on the first try, not even Pulitzer Prize winners. Your first draft is your jumping off point; it's the place where you got all your ideas onto the page in one whole essay. Writing well is always a process; editing and rewriting are endemic to that process.

There are different types of editing, and you can't skimp on any of them if you want a killer personal statement. Sometimes editing is focused on word choice and precision, sometimes on descriptive writing, sometimes on mechanics and punctuation, sometimes on overall flow. This chapter will help you address all these major-editing areas.

Editing is intensive—so much so that the next chapter will be devoted to it as well—but all that effort will result in a statement that will impress program directors and get you residency interviews. Buckle up, this is going to take a lot of work! Hopefully you'll find the process rewarding, but you do need to be prepared for a bit of a long haul. To get an idea of the type of work you'll be doing (and the amount of time required for it), I recommend that you read through this chapter once in full, then go back and work through the exercises.

## REVIEWING YOUR STATEMENT

In the last chapter, I told you to walk away from your personal statement for a while. This is because resting is an important editing pre-step: some of the most successful authors in the world swear by it. In his famed memoir *On Writing*, Stephen King said when he finishes a first draft, he puts it away and doesn't look at it for a minimum of six weeks. You probably don't have six weeks for resting time, but by this point your statement has been sitting in a drawer or tucked away on your computer for at least a few days.

Walking away distanced you from your work both mentally and emotionally; this rest will ultimately make you more productive. The passage of time offers you fresh eyes, a type of impartiality. You'll see your essay for what it is—the good, the bad, and the ugly. You'll be able to make tough editing decisions, decisions that being "too close" to your text would've impeded.

Now that you've let your essay rest, the first step in the editing process is to go back and read what you've written all the way through. Do this without interruption, no matter how many errors you see. Your red pen will get plenty of use soon enough; abstain from wielding it now. Right now, you want to get a sense of your essay as a whole, while being as objective as possible. What are your first impressions? Jot down notes on a separate piece of paper for your own use.

As you read your draft, you may feel panicky if it's not as good as you thought. This is fairly common. Think of your first draft as raw material—a sculptor doesn't go from a block of marble to a detailed statue in one round. From the work you did in the earlier chapters, you know your ideas are solid; all you need now is to bring those ideas to the fore while chipping away at the detritus.

## A TIP FOR TRACKING YOUR EDITS

If your word-processing program allows you to track your changes, turn this feature on now. This will let you see your edited text alongside your original material before you make edits permanent.

If you use the track changes feature, "accept", your changes after each of the exercises in this chapter and then save your document. Alternately, some writers like to save the file with the edits showing, then "accept" the edits before saving this version as a new file.

## SPOT-CHECKING, EIGHT ESSENTIALS

Spot-checking is a way of methodically approaching key elements of your writing and strengthening them. I'm going to outline eight "big" spot-checks in this section, but if you want, you can also address misspellings and obvious grammatical errors in this step, too. You shouldn't be too focused on these things now because fine-tuning comes later—your essay is still changing and evolving—but if you find these types of minor errors distracting, go ahead and correct them as you work. But above all else, be meticulous and thorough as you spot-check. Plan accordingly.

**Spot-check 1:** Your first spot-check focuses on eliminating repeating. In the last chapter, I told you not to worry if you needed to repeat a phrase several times. That was okay for first-draft writing, but now you're editing, and now your focus is different. Go through your essay and eliminate as much literal (or near literal) repeating as you possibly can. ("No repeating" is such a big deal that we'll be revisiting it again later, with a focus on conceptual repeating). As you purge, you may need to smooth over a transition or two; if you can do that easily, go ahead. If not, at least strike through any repeating; let the rest work itself out organically during the editing process.

**Spot-check 2:** Your second spot-check involves revisiting the active and passive voices. You wrote your essay in the active voice, but it's possible that a few passive constructions slipped in there. As you read your statement again, look for any constructions where there's no clear actor nearer to the start of the sentence, as this (broadly speaking) can be an indication of passive-voice construction. With the exception of the "no blame" rule, immediately rewrite any passive sentences. For example, "The instruments were set out by the nurses," becomes, "The nurses set out the instruments," or (if you needed to stress that the nurses did their prep in advance of your arrival), "The nurses had set out the instruments."

**Spot-check 3:** Your third spot check is a sort of ego-check as well. Go through and count the number of times you've used the word *I*, including contractions like *I'd, I'm,* and *I've.* Your statement is about you personally, and so you have to be self-focused to a degree, but you also don't want to sound self-centered. (Hopefully, Spot-check 1 helped you cut out a few uses of *I*; I'm suggesting you pare that number down even further.)

Finding the right number of times to say I is about balance. There's no "perfect" number here; you'll have to use your best judgment. However, if you can edit out a few of your uses, I encourage you to do so. (Tip: One way to do this may be to combine sentences.)

**Spot-check 4:** Your next spot-check requires diving into your thesaurus as you address weak, non-specific, and/or repeated verbs. This process, in itself, is an opportunity to make your writing more visual. Use the richness of the English language to your advantage. If "talked" is in your essay four times, you may be able to change one instance to "chatted," another to "discussed," and a third to "spoke."

**Spot-check 5:** For your fifth spot-check, take a hard look at your descriptions. Are they vivid, do they paint a picture? If a description seems flat, try the following:

Visualize the scene you're trying to convey. Scribble down (on a sheet of paper) words and phrases describing that scene—simple terms like, "blue sky," "small, dark room," or "old wooden clock" will do for the moment. Now open up your thesaurus. Can "blue sky" be more accurately be depicted as "azure horizon?" Is the room you pictured more gloomy than dark, more cramped than small? Is the old clock better described as an antique crafted from walnut? Go through your essay with your new descriptors and insert (or rewrite sentences) as needed, choosing words that will allow the reader to see the image you've visualized. Don't overdo it, though—forced word choices never help. If you, personally, would never use a phrase like "azure horizon," now's not the time to start.

**Spot-check 6:** Shift your focus a bit for your next spot-check. You're applying for a job, remember. This means you need to use some "power" words, like those you'd find on a résumé. You don't want to hammer power words into your writing in awkward ways, but you do want to look for natural opportunities to include:

- Creativity-related words—brainstormed, crafted, designed, developed, formed.

- Deductive-reasoning words—concluded, deduced, determined, diagnosed, inferred.

- Leadership-related words—initiated, managed, orchestrated, ran, supervised.

- Values-related words—compassion, honesty, integrity, loyalty, trustworthiness.

- "You" words (words that hint at your personality)—calm, driven, funny, inquisitive passionate.

**Spot-check 7:** In your seventh spot-check, remove any frivolous words. Here I'm talking about unnecessary modifiers like "most," "rather," "very," and things of this nature. More often than not, these words aren't needed, but if you feel like you've truly lost something without the modifier, open your thesaurus again. Instead of saying "very sad," for example, go for a stronger word like "morose."

While you're checking your modifiers, you'll also be doing another check of your verbs. (Adverbs modify verbs, remember.) As you look at each adverb, examine the verb paired with it. Again find those places where you can substitute more precise language. For example, "smiled widely" could easily become "grinned" or "beamed."

**Spot-check 8:** On your final spot-check, flag any overused words and eliminate or replace them. Words (like *intrinsically*) should appear only once in your essay. If you've used a more common word like *great* seven times, edit until you've reduced that number down to two or three. A limited vocabulary is indicative of poor writing, but worse than that, it reflects a dull, unimaginative author. Unimaginative doesn't describe you: since you've made it this far in your career, you've already proven that you dream big.

These eight essential spot-checks will lead to overall improvement, in ways big and small. Be methodical about them. It may be helpful to think of it as doing triage on your statement—or minor surgery, if you prefer.

By the time you've finished with your spot-checking, your first draft will likely look like a mess, especially if you're using a change-tracking feature. That's okay; each edit is an improvement, and creativity is always (and often wonderfully) messy. We'll begin smoothing things out soon.

**EXERCISE:**

For this exercise, you'll need at least one forty-five-minute writing block to address each of the eight checks outlined above. This equates to six hours of work, but you can take breaks in between and/or spread the process out over two or three days. Focus, patience, and time are your friends as you edit. Don't forget to read through your essay once in full before moving on to spot-checking.

## EXAMINING THE MECHANICS OF YOUR WRITING

The mechanics of your writing is about more than grammar alone—it's also about the structure of your sentences and the flow of your words, among other things. Your edits have likely made your essay a bit choppy, and you've probably created a couple of awkward and/or very wordy sentences, too. This is normal and expected, but you're not trying to present yourself as awkward to program directors. Your writing needs to flow in a natural, forward-movement way. Here are some tips.

**Vary Your Sentence Length:** Read your statement. How many long, winding sentences do you have? While you don't want your essay packed with short, blunt sentences—this will make your writing seem staccato—you don't want lots of complicated sentences that go on for miles, either. (The longer the sentence, the easier it is to screw up the grammar, too.) Unless you're already a strong writer, I suggest a twenty-word rule: If a sentence has more than twenty words, break it up into two sentences, or find a way to trim it down.

There's an additional bonus to the length of your sentences: pieces with varied sentence lengths tend to keep readers more fully engaged.

This could mean good news for you when it comes time for a program director to choose finalists.

**Look Closely at Your Commas:** Commas are tricky, and not even professional writers get them one hundred percent correct all the time. Adding to the complication is that style guides have different rules for comma usage, so there's no one "holy grail of commas" to follow. That said, commas do have a big impact on meaning, clarity, and flow, and so there are some instances where I very much recommend you *always* use them. Let's take a look.

**Introductory Phrases:** Not surprisingly, introductory phrases come at the beginning of sentences. You'll want to follow all introductory phrases with a comma because (generally speaking) this signals to the reader that the subject is coming up in the next part of the sentence.

- After our classes had finished for the day, we went out to dinner.
- Finding the exam room empty, I called to the nurse for assistance.
- To summarize, I have many skills and talents that make me an excellent candidate for this residency.

**The Oxford Comma:** The Oxford (or serial) comma has to do with the way we treat a series of three or more items in a sentence. If there's such a thing as a hot-button grammatical issue, the Oxford comma would be it. On one side of the debate, there are those who all-but swear allegiance to it, while on the other side, many eminently respected publications utterly forbid its use. I'm in the former camp, and you should be too. For reasons I won't get into here, lawsuits have been won and lost over Oxford comma use (or lack thereof), so yes, using it really is important.

In a sentence that contains a series of three or more items, separate each with a comma for clarity and precision.

- My strongest traits are loyalty, compassion, and a positive attitude.

- As I stepped up to the podium, my parents, grandmother, and best friend cheered me on.

- A hug from my father, a kiss from my mother, and a piping-hot traditional dinner greeted me as I arrived home on Thanksgiving Day.

**Nonessential Appositive Phrases:** *Nonessential appositive phrase* is a five-dollar term for a noun phrase that provides "bonus" information about another noun right beside it. (These "bonus" phrases are deemed nonessential largely because pulling them out of your text would still result in a full, grammatically correct sentence.) So, if you wanted your readers to know that you ran into a man named Mr. Crenshaw, *and* you wanted to impart "bonus" info that identifies Mr. Crenshaw as your physics teacher, you could do that using a nonessential appositive phrase, as in the first example below. However, you need commas for clarity.

- I ran into Mr. Crenshaw, my physics teacher, at the park on Saturday.

- I'm applying for this residency on the recommendation of Dr. Sheila Hofstadter, professor of psychiatric medicine.

- Dr. Myers Hurt, author of *Write It*, practices family medicine in Texas.

It's important to use commas with these phrases because program directors read a lot of statements, and along with all that reading comes a bevy of names, titles, awards, and credentials. For directors, all this info can blur together. Help them out by using commas to denote nonessential appositives; it'll aid them in understanding exactly why you're including the "bonus" info. As in the second example above, you want it clear to your reader who Dr. Sheila Hofstadter is, and why her recommendation carries gravitas.

**Eliminate Repeating:** We talked about repeating earlier in this chapter, and we're going to revisit it now because almost all writers repeat in their first draft—it's a byproduct of getting the thoughts in your brain onto the page as quickly as possible. You've already taken out literal repeating, but conceptual repeating is just as problematic. Program directors don't need to be told the same thing two or three times, especially in an essay that's only eight-hundred words. If you've made the same point more than once, now is the time to fine-tune. Choose your most eloquent phrasing and go with that one. Eliminate the others. Even if you feel a point is really, really important and warrants repeating, trust that your audience "heard" you the first time. Because they did.

Keep in mind, however, that part of your conclusion will mirror some part of your introduction. That's a necessary part of an essay's structure and doesn't count as repeating, providing that you restate your point in a fresh way in your conclusion.

You should also note that repeating is different from using *repetition* for effect. For example, if you open your story with a short, vivid phrase, you can *choose* to reuse that phrase. Inten-tional, deliberate repetition is a common device, and it's one that can pack a real wallop. If you've used repetition in your essay, don't edit it out.

---

**EXERCISE:**

For this exercise, you'll need at least one forty-five-minute writing block to address each of the four major mechanical areas outlined above. Feel free to take breaks in between if you need to. Again, focus, patience, and time are your friends as you work. Don't forget to read through your spot-checked essay once in full before examining the mechanics of your writing.

---

**Target Loose Ends with Your Red Pen:** As some general advice, and in no particular order, I also strongly recommend these last few miscellaneous points as targets for your red pen.

- In an essay, always avoid using exclamation points and question marks unless they're absolutely necessary. Both can make you sound unprofessional or immature. If exclamation points exist in your essay, edit them out now. If you can't rewrite sentences with question marks, at the very least make sure you've used your punctuation correctly.

- Reign in your dashes; too many can make your writing sound casual rather than conversational, especially in an essay as brief as eight hundred words. If you've written more than five sentences with dashes, you've likely used too many. Rewrite as needed. It's also a good idea to make sure you haven't used your dashes in close proximity to each other. One dash per single-spaced page is a nice goal.

- Emoji have no place in your personal statement. ASCII will strip these away anyhow, but don't try to get around the encoding with old-school emoticons like this one. :)

- Take out all abbreviations unless they're part of someone's title. ("Dr. Hurt" is okay; "I've wanted to be a dr. my whole life," is not.) Remember that abbreviations are different from acronyms.

Acronyms in the student/medical realm are acceptable and preferable. For example, there's no need to write out "Medical College Admission Test." "MCAT" will do.

- Trim the fat by editing out filler words and phrases. Filler words are those that don't add anything of substance to your writing. They may look pretty, but for the most part you don't need them. Among the most common filler-word culprits are *after that, because of the fact that* (i.e., *because* on its own usually does nicely), *happened to be, next, previously,* and *therefore*. Eliminate these and spackle over the changes if needed. All filler words do is keep your statement from being as crisp and concise as possible.

- If you're writing numbers, pick one format and make sure you've used it consistently throughout your essay. Either write the number out (thirty-three) or use numerals (33). I prefer the former, but you can choose for yourself. Either way, be consistent. Switching between the two will make you seem careless and will be distracting for your audience.

- *It's* versus *its*: This is a sneaky, insidious error that worms its way into almost any draft. When contracted, the two words, *it is* form the word *it's*. However, the adjective meaning "of or relating to it or itself" is *its*. Carefully review each and every usage of both terms.

- Watch your hyphenates: Email or e-mail? Nonessential or non-essential? If you've repeated words with optional hy-phens in your statement, make sure you've written them all in the same way. Small inconsistency issues can make you look unprofessional.

> **EXERCISE:**
> For this exercise, you'll need a one-hour writing block to address the miscellaneous "red pen" targets above. These targets may seem tiny and unimportant, but like most things, your statement is made up of many smaller pieces; if those pieces are jagged, the end product will be rough. Focus as you work, even though this isn't the most exciting part of the process. Break your writing block up into two halves if you need to.

With all this editing, you might be wondering when your second draft will emerge. With your "red pen" work now done, that moment is now: your second draft has just been born. Congratulations! Save your work as a separate file, adding "second draft" to the file name.

———

It's amazing how far you've come! You took your first draft, meticulously worked through *all* of the editing steps I outlined, and now you've arrived at a second draft that's really extraordinary and very "you." You should be proud of yourself. I know I am.

All your writing, editing, and tweaking have stayed private up to this point. That's the way it should be—it can be tough to write your early drafts with someone looking over your shoulder, and early-stage writing time is intentionally cocooned so you can overcome your inner critic as you put your words together. However, now that you have a fully completed second draft, it's time to put your work into the world in a testing-the-waters sort of way.

At this point, you're likely feeling the urge to share your essay with one or two select people; I urge you to take this sharing one step further and embrace feedback to craft your third draft. Looking at your work through the eyes of someone who understands what you're trying to achieve is an invaluable part of the rewriting process.

## SELECTING BETA READERS AND ASKING FOR FEEDBACK

It's natural to want to share your work with others as you move toward completion—it means you're excited about your essay and engaged in the editing process. However, there is such a thing as too many cooks in the kitchen. For this reason, you should reach out to only the five most-qualified people in your circle and ask for their feedback.

Choose your beta readers carefully: your mom already thinks you're special, so unless she's a doctor herself, she almost certainly doesn't have the critical eye you need. By all means, let her read your essay, but do so with the understanding that she can't be one of your beta readers.

The best people to ask for feedback are those who understand the purpose of personal statements as well as the basic requirements for them. If you have former classmates who are currently residents, or if you're lucky enough to know someone who has read a lot of personal statements, their input could be invaluable. You can contact your mentors as well, including professors who've shepherded you along your way these last few years. If someone in your circle is an academic physician or residency program director, definitely reach out to this person. No matter who you ask, make it clear that you're looking for overall first impressions and suggestions for improvement. You're *not* asking for line-by-line editing (That's coming up soon enough!) for spelling and grammar. You need meta-feedback, not micro-editing.

When you approach your beta readers, set a hard deadline for returning comments to you—three or four days, or a week at most. While this may feel a little pushy, I assure you it'll save you a lot of headaches in the long run; a "return by" date will help your selected readers prioritize, and it will give them a sense of how critically important your statement is to you. Additionally, if you choose to give your statement to beta readers outside the world of medicine (which I don't advise, unless you know a professional writer or editor), you should take a minute to explain why you've written your essay and what it's intended to do. Context is key to understanding what you're trying to achieve.

You must accept constructive criticism with an open mind. You may feel a bit hurt by some comments, especially after all the work you've done, but remember that your beta readers took the time to review your essay when they didn't need to. Make it a point to say thank you. And, in a few years, when a graduating med student asks you to read her statement, pay it forward.

Once you have feedback, read the notes provided and look for common threads. If several beta readers mentioned that they were confused at a particular point, that's a good indication that you need to work on this area. However, if one person had an issue with your word choice and four other readers didn't mention it, you can leave it as-is. Sometimes, though, one beta reader will point out something brilliant that all the others missed, and if this happens, the best advice I can give is to simply trust your instinct as you edit further.

---

**EXERCISE:**

For this exercise, you initially don't need a writing block per se, but you do need to select no more than five qualified beta readers and reserve some time for contacting them. (Even in this digital day and age, a phone call—rather than a text, email, or in-app message—when asking for a favor is nice.)

Once you've received back all comments, set aside a thirty-minute writing block to review the feedback and make your own notes. Pay careful attention to your beta readers' suggestions; anything that more than one reader pointed out needs addressing—use your best judgement otherwise.

A day or so later, use a second writing block of at least sixty minutes to revise any problematic areas. If sixty minutes isn't enough time for this very vital step, add additional writing blocks. Work at your own pace.

In addressing your beta readers' concerns, you've now created your third draft. Congratulations! Save your statement as a separate file with "third draft" in the filename.

---

You've done a lot of editing, you've tested the waters, you've gone back and done more editing, and I suspect your personal statement now looks nothing like it did before you began this chapter—both your second and third drafts are now complete!

It's again time for a break. Walk away from your essay for a few days, let your thoughts (and your editing eyes) rest. In the next chapter, you'll have more editing to do, but the heavy lifting is over now. Well done. Stick with me for a few more steps; you're halfway done now!

# CHAPTER 7

## POLISHING YOUR STATEMENT
### ( EDITING, PART II )

After all the heavy changes you've made, and now that you've completed three drafts, you may be wondering what could possibly be left to edit. That's understandable. But as I said earlier, there are different types of editing; these later steps are about polishing, perfecting, and proofreading. Only then will you be ready to begin individualizing your personal statement to specific residency programs.

Now that you've let your statement rest again, it's time to pull it back out and look at it with refreshed eyes. However, this time around, you won't be looking at your content. You'll be looking for the types of smaller errors that can keep a good statement from being great. You *are* pretty great, don't let a few typos stand in your way.

For this chapter, I recommend reading it fully through once, then sitting down to start your polishing.

### CHECKING YOUR GRAMMAR AND SPELLING

I've talked a lot so far about not worrying about your grammar, and even (to some extent) your spelling. I've told you a moment would come when you'd address all that stuff: that moment is now.

I've met a lot of brilliant people who know little about grammar and are terrible at spelling. You may be one of them—but even if you are, your brilliance is no excuse for submitting a personal statement that's full of basic errors. These kinds of mistakes make you look *sloppy* and *amateurish*. I'm sure the words sloppy and amateurish were not two of the adjectives listed in your idea-cloud, so don't blow it now by glossing over the polishing.

It may be helpful to think of the polishing phase like a suit you'll be wearing to an interview. Because you want to present yourself as a professional, you'll have your suit cleaned and well-pressed in advance. A statement that's meticulously polished and proofread is the same type of thing.

English grammar and spelling can be tough for even professional writers. I know authors who still struggle with fundamental things like comma usage and homonyms. This doesn't make them bad writers, but it does mean they need to give special scrutiny to their work before sending it into the world. You're not a professional writer, so you too will need to give your work essay scrutiny.

Extra scrutiny means really drilling down and looking at your statement sentence-by-sentence. Simply running your text through your word-processing program's spellchecker won't be nearly enough: if you accidentally used *their* instead of *they're*, spelling software won't flag the error, because it only looks for misspellings. You'll have to look at each line—and in some cases, each word—with a keen, precise eye. Did you write *vitally* when you meant *vitality*? Now's the time to check.

As for your grammar, the good news is that English in the twenty-first century is arguably more flexible than at any other point in our language's history: you have a lot of leeway in terms of tone, voice, and style. That said, there are still hard-and-fast rules that can't be broken, especially for someone as highly educated as yourself.

The list below contains some areas where the most common grammar errors "hide." I'm not going to define each of these error-types for you—if you need further clarification, a quick Internet search will do—but you should give these points extra attention as you comb through your essay.

- Ambiguous pronouns
- Apostrophes (in both possessives and contractions)

- Capitalization (including proper nouns)
- Consistent Tense (both within a sentence and throughout your essay)
- Dangling participles
- Homonyms and homophones
- Misplaced modifiers
- Subject-verb agreement

---

**EXERCISE:**
Using a ninety-minute writing block, read through your statement line by line and word by word. Go slowly. Examine usages related to each of the bullet points above, but also keep an eye out for typos and other errors.

---

## USING GRAMMAR AND SPELLING TOOLS

If you've gone through your personal statement carefully and you believe there aren't any errors, or if you have no idea what stuff like "dangling participles" and "misplaced modifiers" means and wouldn't know how to spot misuse if it bit you on the nose, don't fret. There are tools that can help you, and everyone (strong writers included) should use them. Because, I promise you, even in an essay you think is perfect, there's a handful of errors (glaring errors included) still in there.

Any writer or editor will tell you that it's incredibly difficult to do a line-by-line edit (Technically called a copyedit) of your own work; proofreaders will tell you the same. One issue with editing your own work is that you're guaranteed to have difficulty separating yourself from your text, which is one of the reasons I've encouraged resting periods.

Resting does help, but it doesn't guarantee you'll catch every error.

By the time you start polishing, you'll have read your statement a dozen times or more—every word will be familiar to you. When you're over-familiar with your writing, your eyes naturally begin to skip over small errors, and this is especially true of unintentionally omitted words. (Our brains are notorious for "filling in" connecting words like a, the, and to when they've accidentally been cut.)

There is good news, however. In this day and age, there are tools that can help you correct your grammar and fix other micro-level errors, and some of these tools are probably already built into your word-processing software. Others are free or low-cost options that will help you achieve your best writing.

If you're using the most recent versions of MS Word, you can turn on the enhanced grammar-checking feature embedded in the program. It's a bit of a hassle to find, but if you open a document and click "File" in the upper left, a new screen pops up. Click "Options" at the bottom, then, in the dialogue box that appears, click "Proofing" on the left. Toward the bottom of the next page, under, "When correcting spelling and grammar in Word," make sure all the boxes are checked, then select "Grammar and Refinements" from the drop-down menu. Once you hit "Recheck Document," common errors in your text will be double underlined for you.

While MS Word's enhanced grammar checker isn't what you'd call world-class, it's a good place to start and will help with the basics. However, the program does get a little confused when it comes to the finer points of grammar, so anytime you see a flagged error, review it carefully before using your own best judgment in terms of correcting. (It's fairly clear when the program is offering you bad advice; I trust you'll be able to spot it easily enough.) Other than that, MS Word's grammar checker can be invaluable.

For those of you using Google Docs, there's a "no fancy settings needed" grammar checker built into the program, but these embedded tools don't rate particularly high on my list. For further refinement, you can download any number of add-ons that will help fill any gaps.

I can't endorse one add-on over the other, though—you'll have to research this yourself.

You can, and should, run your statement through your word processing program's grammar settings, but you should also invest some time into rechecking your text with a program like Grammarly, a popular online tool. Grammarly is perhaps the best-known grammar checker today, and it offers both a free and a paid version. The free version will check your text for basic errors, going a little bit deeper than MS Word or Google Docs, and it will offer you suggestions on how to fix them. It will also tell you if there are high-level grammatical issues in your writing, but you'll have to use the paid version if you want these errors identified individually. Additionally, the paid version offers suggestions on reducing wordiness and use of colloquialisms, and it will propose synonyms if appropriate. Both versions will check your punctuation, flag repeated words (and sometimes repeated short phrases too), catch commonly omitted words, and point out passive voice use.

A word of caution about Grammarly, however. While the program is better than most other online grammar checkers out there (Ginger and Scribens are two others), it's not perfect. Grammarly can sometimes misunderstand where the root of an error lies, and sometimes the fix offered can actually make things worse. Before you click on a suggested "fix," carefully review the flagged error. If the offered solution seems suspicious, reread the sentence and figure out what's wrong for yourself. Also keep in mind that Grammarly is primarily for professional and business writers; it's programmed to follow more strictly-by-the-book grammatical rules than may be necessary for your statement. Use your best judgment.

**EXERCISE:**

Using a forty-five-minute writing block, run your statement through your word processing program's grammar checker. Address any flagged errors.

Once that's done, run your statement through a program like Grammarly and correct again as needed. Remember that no grammar software is perfect (This is precisely the reason you need two different grammar-checking programs.), so use your best judgment when addressing flagged text.

## READING YOUR WORK OUT LOUD

You're so close! Your final draft is emerging, but before you declare your personal statement ready for the next step, read your work aloud, preferably into a recording device. Sitting there talking to yourself might feel awkward at first, but this really is a necessary measure. You've taken my advice so far; humor me for a moment.

Reading a text out loud is a very different experience from reading it silently. It allows you to physically hear your words, which creates a close approximation to how first-time readers will experience them. It will also make some of the most hard-to-catch errors—the stuff that even trained editors have trouble spotting—practically leap off the page.

Using this technique has helped me catch awkward phrases and sentences in my writing. It has also assisted me with identifying overused or repeated words, and it's even helped me detect improper punctuation. If you don't want to read your essay to yourself, you can ask a friend to read it to you, or you can use an app to read it out loud. (MS Word has a "Read Aloud" option on the "Review" menu, which is particularly helpful since you can read along as the program speaks.) No matter how you choose to approach the reading-aloud check, listen carefully: Are their tongue-tying points? Did you type the word *the* twice in a row? Did you omit micro-words like *a, of,* or *to*? Did you refer to a patient in a case study as *obtuse* rather than *obese*?

Reading aloud might seem like a strange approach, but professional writers swear by this trick because it helps them take a step back and experience what they've written in a new way. It engages your aural sensors, not just your visual ones, which means you're feeding your brain the same information in two different ways—a great method for galvanizing your gray matter.

---

**EXERCISE:**

For this exercise, set aside one forty-five-minute writing block. Read your statement aloud or use a text-to-speech app to do it for you. Make note of any awkward-sounding phrases, repeated or overused words, omitted words, and any other errors. Rewrite or correct these as needed.

---

## HIRING A PROFESSIONAL EDITOR

You've done your best with your personal statement, and I commend you for that. However, as I said, it's incredibly difficult to edit and proofread your own writing at this polishing level, and so it's time to reach out to a professional. (Hiring an editor to help you with fine-tuning is very different from paying someone to write or conceptually edit your essay.) At this point, since you've done the hard work—the brainstorming, the writing, the heavy editing, the post-feedback refinements, and this polishing check—it's okay to ask for some professional assistance.

Because polishing-to-precision is so challenging, and because you're not an expert writer or grammarian, I personally recommend hiring a professional even if you think it's an unnecessary expense.

Your statement is the most important piece you've penned thus far, and it's the very thing that could jump-start your career—it's worth *investing* in. Hopefully, with all the work you've already put in, there won't be too much for an editor to do, and therefore the cost will be relatively easy on your wallet. And if there is a lot of work to be done, you'll be better off for having sought professional advice.

Hiring a professional ensures that you'll have a trained set of eyes working to make your best material even better. A good editor will come to your essay without any preconceived notions, and she won't be afraid to gently point out your mistakes. Not only will she be able to catch typos and the typical grammar/spelling stuff, she'll also make clunky sentences flow better, smooth out transitions between sentences or paragraphs, and catch any instances of repeating that you missed. (You'd be surprised how repeating sneaks into an essay!) She will then give your statement a dedicated proofreading pass. By the time your editor is finished, you'll have a letter-perfect document.

In the world of professional editing, the services you need for your essay are most commonly called "copyediting and proofreading;" this is what you need to ask for when approaching an editor. Fortunately, these days, there are many online resources you can use to hire a professional. Here are two I can personally vouch for:

- **Fiverr:** Fiverr is a global online marketplace for freelancers. You'll find the professional services you need under the "Writing & Translation" category.

- **Writer Cartel:** This is a service primarily aimed at marketing/ advertising text, but that may be just what you need. Your statement is part sales pitch, after all.

In addition to these, I've heard good things from others in my circle about:

- **Edit24-7:** This is a site offering fast turn-around times with editors specializing in American English. (Note: Edit24-7 calls the services you need "proofreading and light editing" rather than "copyediting and proofreading.")

- **The Editorial Freelancers Association:** This is a reputable, sizable professional association for freelance editors. Through the EFA's Member Directory, you can find editors specializing in every area under the sun. (My own editor is a member of the EFA.) Additionally, anyone can post a job on the EFA's Job List for free.

- **Freelancer:** This is another online marketplace for freelancers. You can find professionals to help you under the "Writing & Content" category.

- **Upwork:** Upwork may be the largest and most reputable global freelancing marketplace out there, at least as of 2019. You can find editors and proofreaders for hire under the "Writing" category.

## A FEW WORDS OF ADVICE ON USING FREELANCING MARKETPLACES

- Freelancing marketplaces generally use some form of this structure: you post a job, freelancers "bid" on the project, then you select the most promising candidates and interview them before hiring. To facilitate this process, write a job description that's clear but concise, includes your word count, and explicitly states that your essay is a personal statement for a medical residency.

- Remember the adage, "You get what you pay for." When you see editors working for a few dollars per hour or for pennies-on-the-page rates, there's a reason for that. Don't be seduced by the lowest bidders. I'm not saying you need a specialized medical/scientific editor who commands top-tier rates, all I'm saying is that this isn't the time to cheap out.

- On most (if not all) online marketplaces, freelancer profiles include an overall satisfaction rating; comments by past clients are usually available for review as well. Pay strict attention to both of these, especially the client comments. "Disappeared," "late," "missed errors," "non-responsive," and the like do not bode well. While anyone (freelancers or otherwise) can have a bad day or a tough project, a history of non-satisfied clients is a huge red flag.

- It's a good idea to ask freelancers to copyedit, as a sample, the first one-hundred words or so of your essay, just to get a sense of their skill level. Most freelance editors will do this for free as a part of the interview process.

- When interviewing your finalists, opt for a quick phone call/video-chat with each. That way, you can be sure that you're hiring a native English speaker or a certified linguist/translator working professionally in English.

---

**EXERCISE:**

For this exercise, you don't need a writing block per se, but you do need to spend some time visiting the sites listed above. Research costs, freelancer profiles (if applicable), and turn-around times. (If you're going the freelancer route, you'll need extra time for finalist interviews.) Once you've selected the service/freelancer you're most comfortable with, send your essay off for a professional checkup.

---

Wow! look at how far you've come—from your idea-cloud all the way to a professional edit and proofread. You're amazing! With this beautiful essay now in your hands, it's time to tailor it to each residency, and then upload each version to the MyERAS web portal. It won't be long now before you'll begin receiving your first interview requests from program directors.

# CHAPTER 8

## TAILORING YOUR STATEMENT AND UPLOADING IT TO MYERAS

You now have a personal statement that reflects the very best of you—this is no small feat and you should congratulate yourself!

You could simply upload your statement as-is to MyERAS, but I very much encourage you to go one step further. Since MyERAS allows you to upload multiple versions of your statement, you should take the time to tailor your text to each residency you're applying for. By tailoring, I mean adding touches that make it seem as if you custom-wrote your statement for each program. You don't have to go overboard, but subtle changes can go a long way in establishing individual reader rapport.

You must make these tailoring-changes deliberately and carefully, since your statement has already been professionally proofread. Take your time and work slowly—now isn't the moment to introduce new errors into your otherwise letter-perfect essay. You'll do just fine, though, if you follow the steps I outline in this last chapter. As in the other editing-related chapters, you should read through this chapter once, then do the work described.

At this point, I bet the thought of doing further work on your essay makes you want to run away screaming. I don't blame you. But you really are in the home stretch now; hang in there!

### THE BENEFITS OF CUSTOM-TAILORING YOUR STATEMENT

Tailoring your personal statement might seem like a waste of time, especially since you've already invested so much effort, but there are two main benefits to doing this extra bit of work, and they both speak to a powerful, fundamental aspect of the human condition: making connections. Take the word of someone who's read thousands of residency essays—when an applicant can speak to her readers about very-specific shared goals, experiences, or locales, readers *want* to pay that much more attention. Sparking this kind of interest goes further than general reader engagement; it forges an immediate writer-reader bond.

As your essay is now, it'll be just one in the sea of dozens, if not hundreds, of statements that any given program director needs to read this year alone. Essays that include specific references to a director's program, hospital, or city are instantly going to pique her interest. By evidencing even a small (but sincere!) personal link in your essay, the director will feel a connection to your writing and, by extension, to you. This connection, in itself, may be enough to get your entire application moved into the "further consideration" pile. If your application is in the "further consideration" pile, it's also *out* of the rejection pile, which means you've got your foot in the door!

Secondly, if you include points about the program itself, you're tapping into the pride that a director takes in her work, and you're indicating that you share common goals and visions. Very few medical professionals go to work each day utterly despising what they do and the institution they work for; for everyone else, they take an active interest in making their programs the best they can be. In tailoring your statement, you're signaling that you respect their work and want to be a part of those good efforts. After all, humans are social creatures, and we enjoy working with those who share our interests and passions.

These are two major, powerful benefits you can reap with just a few minutes of extra work per application. It's worth the effort. At the very least, it's worth it for your top-five residency programs.

## TAILORING POINTS

As you begin to tailor, the basics are the first thing you'll want to address. The points below are all public information; if you don't have this info already, a quick Internet search will get you what you need. List the residencies you're applying for on a separate sheet of paper and write these details out. That way, you won't get confused as you work.

- The program director's name and name of the program
- The hospital/clinic/center housing the program
- The city and state of the program
- The specific residency position
- "Big name" doctors in the program who you would like to work with or study under (if applicable)

As you insert this info, *highlight your changes*. This is essential. (You'll see why in a moment.) It's also essential to title each tailored file properly—and with an obvious file name—so you can upload it to MyERAS without difficulty or confusion. Example: "Personal statement, Houston Methodist, obstetrics residency."

---

**EXERCISE:**

Reserve one thirty-minute writing bock to gather the public information outlined above for each of your top-five residency positions. List these facts on a separate piece of paper.

Use five more fifteen-minute writing blocks to insert tailoring details where appropriate, highlighting your changes as you work. Go one residency at a time. Save each version of your statement as a new file with an obvious file name.

Tip: keep no more than two files open at any given time— the original version, and one tailored version.

---

## MICRO-TAILORING

There are other tiny touches you can make to tailor your personal statement even further to a specific residency. Maybe the program you're applying to is in a city you remember fondly, or maybe the hospital that houses it has a mission you'd be particularly proud to support. Perhaps you're applying to a residency based in a small, regional hospital and you have a passion for rural healthcare. Whatever it is, if you can add a few words here or there (Subtle changes only, please!) expressing your interest and personal connection, you should.

To help you organize your micro-tailoring thoughts, make a list on sheet of paper idea-cloud style. Write down everything that's special about each individual residency, along with everything that contributed to your decision to apply to it. Location, hospital reputation, mentoring programs, specialized procedures, specific doctors working in the department, and much more are all fair game.

Once you've collected your thoughts, it should be fairly easy to slip these details into your essay. Don't overdo this level of tailoring, and make these changes very, very carefully. Don't forget to highlight your edits as you work.

It's crucial that you add the right information to the right version of your statement, and that you make any such changes *thoroughly and completely throughout*. For example, if you're applying to residencies in, say, Boston and Los Angeles, you wouldn't want—somewhere in the middle of your LA version—to accidentally imply that UCLA Medical Center is on the east coast. Be careful and thorough as you tailor.

---

**EXERCISE:**

Using a thirty-minute writing block, make an idea-cloud-type capturing everything you feel connects you in a personal way to each of your top five residencies. (If you only have a personal connection to, say, three of your top five programs, don't sweat it. Focus on these three only; don't "force" connections that you don't truly feel.)

For each statement where you have micro-tailoring to add, reserve one thirty-minute writing block. Insert these details where appropriate. Work slowly and highlight your changes as you go. Use extra caution to ensure all edits are logical, flow well, and are free from typos or other errors. Save and close all versions of your statement.

Go back and review each micro-tailored document to make sure your changes accurately reflect each institution/residency.

Tip: Keep only one version of your statement open at a time as you review.

## ONE LAST CHECK

You've done awesome. Walk away from your essay—all versions of it—for at least twenty-four hours before doing this one last check. (Yes, this check *is* really necessary; no you can't skip it; and yes, I'm sorry.)

**EXERCISE, PART I:** After resting for at least twenty-four hours, print out the original, non-tailored version of your personal statement in hard copy. Using a ruler to guide you, proofread your essay one last time word-by-word and line-by-line. If you find an error, return to your computer and meticulously correct it across *all* versions of your statement. This step should take about thirty minutes.

**EXERCISE, PART II:** Print out all tailored versions of your essay. Using a ruler to guide you, proofread each version, looking at the highlighted text only. Return to your computer and correct typos or other errors as needed. This step should take about thirty minutes.

**EXERCISE, PART III:** Now open up each of your electronic files and *remove the highlighting across all versions* of your statement. Save these as new files marked with FINAL on the end of the filename. These are the versions you'll be uploading to MyERAS. Delete older versions or move them to a dedicated subfolder. This step should take about fifteen minutes.

## SUBMITTING YOUR STATEMENT VIA MyERAS

Wow, you're good! You now have a finished, polished, and proofread personal statement—in various tailored versions—ready to submit with your ERAS application. This is the moment you've been working toward all these pages; this is the *career* you've been working toward all these years. I don't have much more guidance to offer, except for a couple of quick tips about MyERAS.

One of the things I like best about MyERAS is that you can save multiple versions of your statement/application. I encourage you to upload each tailored version of your statement with one caveat: you must double- and triple-check to ensure you are uploading the correct version to each application. As with all uploads/attachments, it's frustratingly easy to make a mistake. Sending a program the wrong version of your essay will surely take you out of the running for that position.

In MyERAS, you can preview your uploaded statements as PDF files. Review these. The main benefit of previewing the PDFs is that you can see each document in exactly the same way as your readers will—any odd spacing, weird formatting, or extra indentations at paragraph breaks will all show up. To open the preview, choose "View/

Print MyERAS Application," which is located in the "Application" section of the dashboard at the top-right of each page. If you see a formatting glitch, you can return to your document, find the culprit behind the issue, and then re-upload your essay before finishing the application process.

Yes, you read that correctly: finishing the application process. Go ahead and click "Submit." You've made it, you're DONE! Great work!

Congratulations! You're now on your way to Matching in the perfect residency for you! You stuck with me through this whole process, and together we've crafted a personal statement that tells program directors who you are as a person, professional, and potential colleague. You've told your story, and you've told it well.

One last piece of advice: now's the time to treat yourself—certainly you've earned a night out. Enjoy yourself for a little while. Then sit back and watch as your interview requests begin pouring in. By this time next year, you'll be a practicing physician!

# A CLEAN BILL OF HEALTH
## ( A FAREWELL FROM THE AUTHOR )

Thank you for reading *Write It*. The Match system is highly competitive, but I'm confident that the information and exercises included in this workbook have given you a true edge. By now, I'm sure you're well on your way to landing your first residency interview.

Writing your personal statement wasn't easy, but because you put so much extra effort into your essay, your application will stand out. An eye-catching statement like yours ensures that more program directors will invite you to interview. Whatever your specialty or area(s) of interest, more interviews mean more chances to shine!

I wish you good luck with your job search. I'm certain that you'll soon be happily employed in the residency program that's perfect for you.

# GLOSSARY OF SPECIALIZED ACRONYMS & TERMS

**ACGME (Accreditation Council for Graduate Medical Education):**
The ACGME, a non-profit council, accredits the majority of graduate medical training programs for US physicians, including residency and internship programs.

**COMLEX (Comprehensive Osteopathic Medical Licensing Examination):**
COMPLEX is a national, three-tiered, standardized-licensure exam. COMLEX is similar to the USMLE (See below.) but is specifically designed for those pursuing careers in osteopathic medicine.

**ERAS (Electronic Residency Application Service):**
ERAS is a web-based service, provided and maintained by the Association of American Medical Colleges, that standardizes and streamlines the residency application process in the US. By using ERAS, prospective residents can build and send their application(s) and supporting materials to residency programs.

**Match, The:**
The Match is a nickname for the National Resident Matching Program. (See below.) This program pairs graduating medical students with residency positions at teaching hospitals.

*Match* is also used to denote positions open in this program. (e.g. She was highly interested in three available Matches.) *Match Day* refers to the dedicated day when applicants are informed of their Matches.

In verb form, *Match* refers to placement or anticipated placement in a residency via the National Resident Matching Program. (e.g., She Matched with a program in an urban hospital.)

**MCAT (Medical College Admission Test):**
   The MCAT is a standardized exam used throughout North America for prospective medical students. A solid MCAT score is a requirement for admission into most US medical schools.

**MyERAS (My Electronic Residency Application Service):**
   MyERAS is a part of the ERAS system. The web page at which a prospective resident creates a profile and subsequently submits residency applications is called MyERAS.

**NRMP (National Resident Matching Program):**
   The National Resident Matching Program is a non-profit, non-governmental organization in the US that places graduating medical students into residency programs.

**SOAP (Supplemental Offer and Acceptance Program):**
   For those who do not initially Match, SOAP gives eligible applicants a second chance, immediately following Match Day, to be paired with a residency position.

**USMLE (United States Medical Licensing Examination):**
   The USMLE is a three-step standardized test required in the US for medical licensure. A medical student's score on the USMLE Step 1 is the most-heavily-weighted component of a residency application.

# ACKNOWLEDGMENTS

I would like to first thank the medical students I teach—past, present, and future. You are my primary inspiration for this text, and you constantly drive me to better myself as a physician.

Thank you to my editor, Erika DeSimone, for taking my ideas and turning them into something legible. Your efforts created a product that I am proud to put my name on.

Last but certainly not least, I owe many thanks to my wife Ragan, who listens to all of my harebrained ideas patiently, and whose infinite understanding keeps my writing alive. Ragan, without you, none of this would be possible.

# ABOUT THE AUTHOR

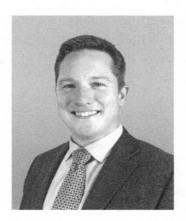

Dr. Myers R. Hurt III is an author, entrepreneur, and board-certified physician. As a graduating medical student, he secured his first-choice Match at the University of Texas Medical Branch in Galveston. During his last year in the program, he served as chief resident. Dr. Hurt then joined the faculty of the Department of Family Medicine as an assistant professor, where he split his time between medical education and clinical practice. He remains passionate about helping emerging doctors find their own paths to success.

Dr. Hurt currently writes a biweekly health column for *The Paris News* in Texas. His articles have appeared in the *Medical Journal–Houston, Explore: The Journal of Science & Healing, the Daily News* (Galveston, TX), and the Student Doctor Network. His previous speaking engagements have included guest lectures at the Osher Lifelong Learning Institute at the University of Texas Medical Branch, the Society of Teachers of Family Medicine, the Texas Academy of Family Physicians, and the University of Miami's School of Nursing.

His first book, *Getting In: How to Stand Out from the Crowd and Ace Your Residency Interview*, has sold thousands of copies and consistently reaches #1 in Amazon's Medical Education category during the residency-interview season. His podcast, "Countdown to the MATCH," has seen over 20,000 unique downloads across a variety of platforms.

Dr. Hurt is a board-certified family practice provider, as well as a board-certified integrative holistic medicine provider. He is currently in private family-practice in Paris, Texas. He blogs regularly at his site, www.DrMyersHurt.com.

Made in the USA
Las Vegas, NV
12 November 2021